Insights Into Algae - Fundamentals, Culture Techniques and Biotechnological Uses of Microalgae and Cyanobacteria

Edited by Ihana Aguiar Severo, Walter J. Martínez-Burgos and Juan Ordonez

Published in London, United Kingdom

Insights Into Algae - Fundamentals, Culture Techniques and Biotechnological Uses of Microalgae and Cyanobacteria
http://dx.doi.org/10.5772/intechopen.1001726
Edited by Ihana Aguiar Severo, Walter J. Martínez-Burgos and Juan Ordonez

Contributors
Antonio Idà, Ashar Khalil, Borut Lazar, Davide Carecci, Dijana Lalić, Elena Ficara, Eleonora Sforza, Gabriel Dylan Scoglio, Giorgos Markou, Ihana Aguiar Severo, Ioannis Tzovenis, Juan Carlos Ordonez, Leonardo Pattaro, Maja Berden Zrimec, Nabil Al-Shwafi, Narcís Ferrer-Ledo, Roberta Pozzan, Robert Reinhardt, Saida A. Dowman, Sameera Y. Al-Hakmi, Seyed Mojtaba Soleymani Robati, Silvio Mangini, Sophia Papadaki, Stefano Canziani, Stefano Scoglio, Walter José Martínez-Burgos

First published in London, United Kingdom, 2024 by IntechOpen
IntechOpen is the global imprint of INTECHOPEN LIMITED, registered in England and Wales, registration number: 11086078, 167-169 Great Portland Street, London, W1W 5PF, United Kingdom

British Library Cataloguing-in-Publication Data
A catalogue record for this book is available from the British Library

Additional hard and PDF copies can be obtained from orders@intechopen.com

Insights Into Algae - Fundamentals, Culture Techniques and Biotechnological Uses of Microalgae and Cyanobacteria
Edited by Ihana Aguiar Severo, Walter J. Martínez-Burgos and Juan Ordonez
p. cm.
Print ISBN 978-0-85466-845-8
Online ISBN 978-0-85466-844-1
eBook (PDF) ISBN 978-0-85466-846-5

For EU product safety concerns:
IN TECH d.o.o., Prolaz Marije Krucifikse Kozulić 3, 51000 Rijeka, Croatia,
info@intechopen.com or visit our website at intechopen.com.

Meet the editors

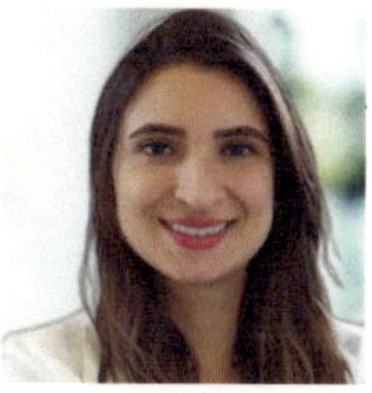

Dr. Ihana Aguiar Severo is a researcher at the Center for Advanced Power Systems (CAPS), Florida State University, USA. She also collaborates as a researcher at the Sustainable Energy Research and Development Center (NPDEAS), Federal University of Paraná, Brazil. She holds a Ph.D. and a master's degree in food science and technology (Federal University of Santa Maria, Brazil). In addition, Dr. Severo has experience in food science and technology with a focus on microalgal biotechnology. Her scientific and technological research interests include microalgae-based processes and products, photobioreactors, process integration, renewable energy, and environmental sustainability.

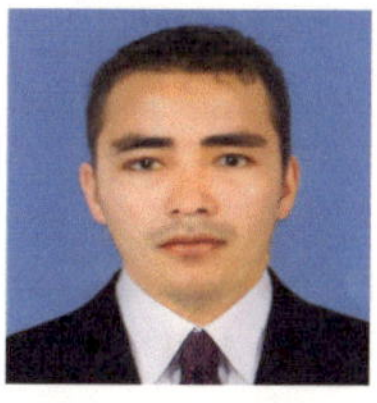

Dr. Walter Jose Martinez Burgos is a researcher in the postgraduate program in bioprocess engineering and biotechnology at the Federal University of Paraná (UFPR) in Brazil, where he has developed research with bacteria, yeasts, filamentous fungi, and microalgae. He holds a master's degree in environmental engineering (Universidad del Norte, Barranquilla-Colombia) and a Ph.D. in bioprocess engineering and biotechnology (UFPR, Curitiba-Brazil), with a degree in food engineering (Universidad de Cordoba, Monteria-Colombia). Dr. Martinez has extensive experience in optimization, scale-up, and product development using microorganisms and microbial enzymes.

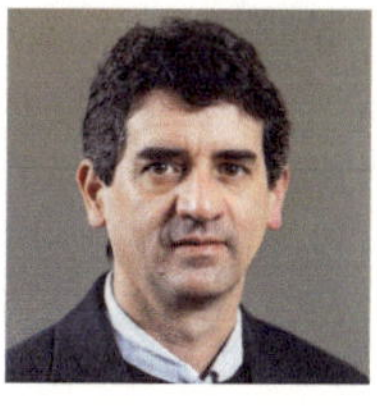

Dr. Juan C. Ordonez is a full professor in the Department of Mechanical Engineering, FAMU-FSU College of Engineering, Florida A&M University, Florida State University; the director of the Energy and Sustainability Center (ESC); and the principal investigator in the Thermal Modeling and Management Group at the Center for Advanced Power Systems (CAPS). His research interests include renewable energy systems, thermodynamic optimization, heat transfer, constructal theory, thermal management and modeling of energy systems, fuel cells, and design and optimization of microalgae photobioreactors.

Contents

Preface

The field of algal biotechnology has witnessed remarkable advancements over the past few decades, driven by the urgent need for sustainable and renewable resources. *Insights into Algae – Fundamentals, Culture Techniques, and Biotechnological Uses of Microalgae and Cyanobacteria* aims to capture the depth of this exciting domain, providing a comprehensive overview of the fundamental concepts, culture techniques, and biotechnological applications of these versatile microorganisms.

Algae, which include both microalgae and cyanobacteria, although they have different biological characteristics, are crucial to many ecological and industrial processes. Microalgae are eukaryotic organisms, while cyanobacteria are prokaryotic. Still, both share the extraordinary ability to thrive in a wide variety of environments and to convert solar energy into chemical energy through photosynthesis. This ability allows them to play a critical role in bioremediation, wastewater treatment, and carbon dioxide capture to address pressing environmental challenges. In addition, algae contribute to energy production, environmental sustainability, and food security.

This book explores the myriad benefits of algae, from their economic value in the commercial sector to their potential to produce biomass to meet the growing global demand for renewable resources. It also covers culture techniques, operational strategies for microalgae and cyanobacteria cultivation, and environmental applications.

As the specialized market for algal bioprocesses and bioproducts continues to expand, this book highlights research and technological advances that promise to revolutionize the field. Therefore, this book is a compendium that will be valuable to anyone interested in algae's scientific and practical aspects, from basic research to applied technologies and commercial uses.

We would like to thank all the contributors and collaborators who made this project possible.

Ihana Aguiar Severo and Juan Ordonez
Florida State University,
USA

Walter José Martínez-Burgos
Federal University of Paraná (UFPR),
Brazil

Chapter 1

Introductory Chapter: Cyanobacteria – An Overview

Walter José Martínez-Burgos, Roberta Pozzan, Ihana Aguiar Severo and Juan Carlos Ordonez

1. Introduction

Cyanobacteria are prokaryotic organisms that can be found in the most diverse ecosystems [1]. When first discovered, cyanobacteria were considered to be plant-like organisms, due to their photosynthetic nature, and were then named "Schizophyceae," "Cyanophyta," "Cyanophyceae," or "blue-green algae." Because they are prokaryotic organisms, the term "cyanobacteria" was also used [2].

Although in the past, only bacteria that perform oxygenated photosynthesis were considered cyanobacteria, recent metagenomic studies demonstrate that the group of cyanobacteria also includes certain species of non-photosynthetic bacteria [3]. In this chapter, however, we primarily consider photosynthetic cyanobacteria for discussion purposes.

1.1 General characteristics

Cyanobacteria do not have internal cell membranes that delimit the cell nucleus from other organelles and are therefore classified as prokaryotic organisms, which microscopically distinguishes them from algae, microalgae, and plants. They can be found as unicellular, colonial, or multicellular organisms and inhabit the most diverse environments; they can be planktonic (suspended in water), benthic (attached to surfaces), or metaphytic (attached to macrophytes or other surfaces submerged in water) [4].

They are photosynthetic organisms and therefore have a pigment called chlorophyll-a. However, due to the absence of internal cell membranes, cyanobacteria do not have chloroplasts, and, therefore, chlorophyll is found inside simple thylakoids, where light-dependent photosynthetic reactions take place. Cyanobacteria also have carotenoids (whose main function is photoprotection) and accessory pigments, such as phycobilins (e.g., phycocyanin and phycoerythrin), which do more than provide the characteristic cyanobacterial color: phycocyanins and phycoerythrins absorb some wavelengths of active radiation and transfer the absorbed light energy to chlorophyll-a in photosystem II [5].

Cyanobacteria reproduce by asexual reproduction, the division of vegetative cells. In unicellular species, cells divide completely, and some can form colonies, an aggregate of single cells in a mucilaginous matrix. When their cell division occurs in a single plane, they can form pseudofilaments, linear colonies formed by unicellular cyanobacteria. In true filamentous cyanobacteria, the cells remain connected after division, forming structures called trichomes or filaments. The filaments divide through a single plane of division that can also project in multiple directions, forming false-branched filaments, or they can divide through multiple planes of cell division, forming true-branched filaments [6].

The cellular morphology of these organisms is quite diverse and can be used to identify different species and taxonomic groups. The cell shape of cyanobacteria can be spherical, ellipsoid, cylindrical, conical, or discoid. Their size also varies greatly, from the so-called picobacteria, spherical cyanobacteria with a very small cell diameter (0.2 μm), to filamentous forms that can reach up to a few millimeters [7].

Despite not having flagella, many cyanobacteria have mobility mechanisms, although they are not very well elucidated. In fact, some filamentous species can develop hormogonia, reproductive and mobile units, which are formed by the fragmentation of filaments and then released from the parental filament. Hormogonia perform gliding movements until they develop into a new trichome [8].

Some specialized cellular structures are also found in some cyanobacterial species. Aerotopes, for example, are structures formed by cylindrical proteins that form air vesicles. These vesicles are filled with air, which diffuses into their interior, making the cyanobacterial cells less dense than water and allowing them to float or emerge. Aerotopes are refractory to light in microscopy techniques and are therefore used to differentiate taxa in microscopic analyses [9].

Not only specialized cellular structures can be identified in cyanobacteria, but there are also entire specialized cells that are morphologically distinct from vegetative cells, such as heterocytes and akinetes cells. The first are cells that enable nitrogen fixation, a process called diazotrophy, where nitrogenase enzymes reduce nitrogen to ammonium; therefore, heterocytes have an extra cell envelope to maintain the cell interior in anoxic conditions, and they do not have a complete photosynthetic mechanism, as this could damage nitrogenases with the production of oxygen. Akinetes are spore-like cells, larger than vegetative cells, with a multilayered cell wall and glycogen and cyanophycin granules. In general, the formation of heterocytes and akinetes is closely related to environmental conditions [10].

1.2 Taxonomy of cyanobacteria

The criteria for classifying cyanobacteria are phylogenetic relationships that indicate their grouping into taxa that share a common evolutionary ancestor, as is the case for all other living organisms. Initially, the taxonomic classification of cyanobacteria, as well as several other organisms, was based solely on morphological characteristics, that is, cellular properties observed through microscopic techniques. However, molecular techniques are now being used to elucidate the correct taxonomy of species, including cyanobacteria. Thus, many classifications have been revised, regrouped, and even renamed, and many of them are probably not definitive and may change as more research is carried out at the molecular level [11].

There is no precise definition of species for the taxonomic classification of cyanobacteria, as this would require obtaining pure, axenic cultures, which is very difficult in the case of cyanobacteria. Furthermore, there are two different nomenclature systems for these organisms: the International Code of Nomenclature for Algae, Fungi, and Plants (ICN) and the International Code of Nomenclature for Bacteria (ICNB). Thus, depending on the scientific vision and knowledge of the taxonomist, a given species can be identified in different ways, confusing the literature [3]. Some authors argue that the description of cyanobacterial taxa would be more appropriate using the bacteriological code since it is already known that cyanobacteria are a monophyletic branch in the bacterial phylogenetic tree [2].

2. Biotechnological applications of cyanobacteria

Cyanobacteria have attracted considerable research attention due to their versatility in various applications, including energy (e.g., biodiesel, biohydrogen, biogas, and bioethanol), pharmaceuticals, food additives, and fertilizers. They are used in bioremediation processes such as wastewater treatment and CO_2 capture [4]. **Figure 1** illustrates the multiple uses of cyanobacteria in the industrial sector.

2.1 Bioenergy

The depletion of the world's oil reserves and the environmental impact caused by the emission of polluting gases during fuel combustion have forced humanity to look for sustainable energy alternatives [12–14]. Cyanobacteria emerge as a promising energy source, primarily due to their significant lipid accumulation potential, which can subsequently be converted into biodiesel through transesterification [15]. Furthermore, cyanobacteria have high growth rates, high photosynthetic capacity, low nutritional requirements, and do not need fertile land. However, its growth and lipid accumulation are affected by several factors, such as light intensity, temperature, pH of the medium, the availability of macro and micronutrients in the medium, and cultivation systems, such as closed photobioreactors or open raceway ponds [16].

The concentrations of phosphorus and nitrogen are decisive in the accumulation of lipids by cyanobacteria, which can accumulate up to 50% of their weight in lipids. For example, the cyanobacterium *Microcystis protocystis* accumulated around 42% of its weight in lipids under controlled nitrogen and phosphorus conditions. Other

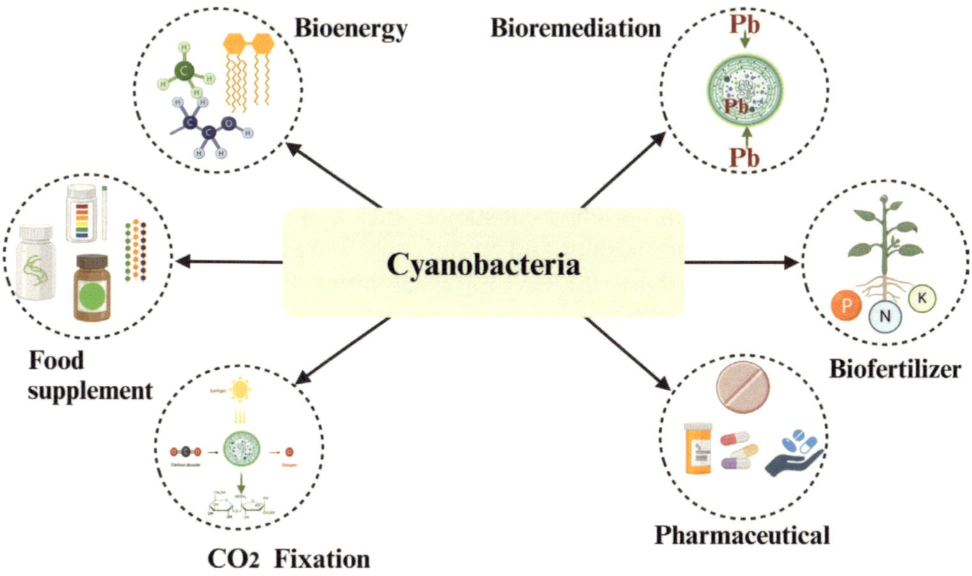

Figure 1.
Applications of cyanobacteria.

cyanobacteria, such as *Synechocystis* sp. PCC 6803 and *Synechococcus elongatus*, can accumulate up to 20% of lipids of their weight [15].

On the other hand, cyanobacteria can also be used to produce high-energy molecules such as ethanol. For example, Dexter & Fu [17] developed a mutant cyanobacterium *Synechocystis* sp. PCC 6803 that can photoautotrophically convert CO_2 into bioethanol. The transformation was carried out using a double homologous recombination system to integrate the genes for pyruvate decarboxylase (pdc) and alcohol dehydrogenase II (adh) from the obligate ethanol-producing *Zymomonas mobilis* into the cyanobacterial chromosome. Thus, Liang et al. [18] used a *Synechocystis* PCC 6803 mutant to achieve ethanol concentrations of up to 900 mg/L ethanol.

Cyanobacteria can also produce other energetic molecules, such as methane (CH_4). According to Bižić et al. [19], some cyanobacteria living in marine, freshwater, and terrestrial environments produce methane at substantial rates under light, dark, oxic, and anoxic conditions.

2.2 Biofertilizer

The frequent application of chemical or synthetic nitrogen-based fertilizers changes the composition and structure of the soil, in addition to negatively affecting the microbial flora [20–22]. Therefore, nitrogen sources that are less aggressive to the environment are needed. One of the alternatives is biological nitrogen fixation, which is a process generally developed by microorganisms that convert atmospheric or inorganic nitrogen into a form of nitrogen that can be used by plants. According to Rashid et al. [23], employing nitrogen-fixing microorganisms presents an economically appealing and environmentally friendly alternative. Among the various microorganisms capable of fixing atmospheric nitrogen, cyanobacteria are particularly noteworthy.

Cyanobacteria are considered one of the most promising microorganisms for sustainable agricultural development due to their high nitrogen fixation capacity. According to Joshi et al. [21] and Song et al. [24], cyanobacteria such as *Diazotrophs* are potentially useful microorganisms for the production of biofertilizers. Cyanobacteria such as *Anabaenas* can fix up to 60 kg of atmospheric nitrogen/ha in the soil. Other microorganisms such as *Anabaena variabilis* and *Nostoc linkia* also have a significant ability to fix nitrogen at around 25 kg nitrogen/hectare [21].

According to Song et al. [24], cyanobacteria play an essential role in maintaining and improving soil fertility, due to which these microorganisms contribute to the formation of porous soils and produce substances such as phytohormones (auxiana and gibberellins), as well as vitamins and amino acids that promote plant growth. Furthermore, cyanobacteria also improve water retention capacity due to their gelatinous structure [21, 25, 26].

2.3 Food supplement and pharmaceutical products from cyanobacteria

Cyanobacteria are considered foods and dietary supplements because they are a source of carbohydrates, proteins, peptides, essential amino acids, fibers, lipids, polyunsaturated fatty acids, minerals, vitamins, etc., compounds necessary for human and animal nutrition [27]. Some of these compounds have antioxidant, antimicrobial, anticancer, antimycotic, and antifungal properties, among others [28].

Some species of *Spirulina* are important sources of macromolecules, including mainly proteins. They have been sold as natural products, spreading worldwide popularity for being one of the most nutritious foods from an alternative source. *Spirulina* has the outstanding ability to accumulate protein and has already been used in meat substitutes, food products, animal feed, nutraceuticals, and pharmaceuticals [27].

Ahmed [29] evaluated the antimicrobial activity of methanolic strata of cyanobacteria such as *Oscillatoria formosa*, *Nostoc caeruleum*, *Cylindrospermum majus*, and *Spirulina platensis* against the bacteria *Staphylococcus aureus, Escherichia coli*, *Klebsiella pneumoniae*, *Pseudomonas aeruginosa* and the fungi *Trichophyton mentagrophytes*, *Candida albicans*, and *Aspergillus fumigatus.* The results obtained showed that the alcoholic extract of *S. platensis* was the most effective against the microorganisms tested.

According to Vijayakumar & Menakha [30], cyanobacteria are also sources of bioactive secondary metabolites such as apratoxins, lynbyabellin, and curacin A, compounds that can be used to manufacture drugs against complex diseases such as cancer. Some freshwater cyanobacteria produce peptides with side chains that are effective against different enzymes such as microginin, aeruginosin, anabaenopeptin, etc. [31].

Additionally, bioactive compounds from some species of cyanobacteria have been explored for biomedical purposes. Polysaccharides are interesting sources due to their many physicochemical properties and biological roles. These biomolecules, especially exopolysaccharides, are extremely important for market purposes because they can be used as anti-inflammatory, immunomodulatory, antiglycemic, antitumor, antioxidant, anticoagulant, antilipidemic, antiviral, antibacterial and antifungal agents [32].

2.4 Cyanobacteria in bioremediation processes

Cyanobacteria play a significant role in bioremediation processes due to their unique capabilities. Bioremediation involves the use of living organisms to detoxify and eliminate pollutants from the environment. These microorganisms contribute to the biogeochemical cycles of carbon and nitrogen [31, 33]. Furthermore, cyanobacteria are potent bioremediation agents due to their ability to grow under extreme conditions and metabolize different metabolites. Compounds that have been bioremediated with cyanobacteria include pesticides, heavy metals, paints, and emerging contaminants such as hormones, pharmaceuticals, and others [31].

One of the most important xenobiotics removed by cyanobacteria are heavy metals such as Mn, Zn, Cu, Cd, and Pb. Some species of cyanobacteria can produce exopolysaccharides that are used to sequester xenobiotics [34, 35]. According to Potnis et al. [35], biofilms produced by *Phormidium* can sequester up to 99% Cu ions. Biofilms of *Nostoc commune* and *Nostoc linckia* can remove between 55% and 87% [36].

Cyanobacteria are utilized in the treatment of various types of wastes. They can effectively reduce organic pollutants and nutrients in wastewater, contributing to the purification of water before it is released back into natural ecosystems. In addition, cyanobacteria can fix carbon dioxide through photosynthesis. This capability is harnessed not only for potential biofuel production but also for CO_2 capture purposes. By converting CO_2 into organic matter, cyanobacteria can help mitigate greenhouse gas levels in the atmosphere [4].

3. Final remarks

The diversity of important applications of cyanobacteria in numerous technological production routes makes these microorganisms biocatalysts with a broad potential for industrial exploitation. Despite this potential, in the current scenario, the competition with consolidated technological routes based on non-renewable fossil inputs makes cyanobacteria-based processes economically unfeasible. In this way, new industrial approaches have been proposed and implemented to effectively enable the technical-economic success of cyanobacterial processes. The integration and intensification of processes associated with the biorefinery concept have been considered the main engineering strategies that will allow broad commercial exploitation of these microorganisms. These technological routes are oriented toward the effective use of industrial resources based on more efficient equipment, material flows (e.g., effluents), and processing techniques. Finally, continued research into their biology and exploration of their unique capabilities offer promising avenues for addressing environmental sustainability challenges in various industries.

Author details

Walter José Martínez-Burgos[1], Roberta Pozzan[2], Ihana Aguiar Severo[3,4]* and Juan Carlos Ordonez[4]

1 Department of Bioprocess Engineering and Biotechnology, Polytechnic Center, Federal University of Paraná (UFPR), Curitiba, PR, Brazil

2 Department of Cell Biology, Laboratory of Cell Toxicology, Federal University of Paraná (UFPR), Curitiba, PR, Brazil

3 Sustainable Energy Research and Development Center (NPDEAS), Federal University of Paraná (UFPR), Curitiba, PR, Brazil

4 Department of Mechanical Engineering, FAMU-FSU College of Engineering, Energy and Sustainability Center, Center for Advanced Power Systems (CAPS), Florida A&M University, Florida State University, Tallahassee, FL, United States

*Address all correspondence to: is23@fsu.edu; ihana.aguiar@gmail.com

References

[1] Sukharevich VI, Polyak YM. Global occurrence of Cyanobacteria: Causes and effects (Review). Inland Water Biology. 2020;**13**(4):566-575. DOI: 10.1134/S1995082920060140

[2] Vidal L, Ballot A, et al. Introduction to cyanobacteria. In: Toxic Cyanobacteria in Water. 2nd ed. Vol. 1. Abington, OX: CRC Press; 2021. pp. 163-212

[3] Kaštovský J. Welcome to the jungle!: An overview of modern taxonomy of cyanobacteria. Hydrobiologia. 2023;**851**:1063-1077. DOI: 10.1007/s10750-023-05356-7

[4] Zahra Z, Choo DH, Lee H, Parveen A. Cyanobacteria: Review of current potentials and applications. Environments – MDPI. 2020a;**7**(2):1-17. DOI: 10.3390/environments7020013

[5] Pagels F, Pereira RN, Vicente AA, Guedes AC. Extraction of pigments from microalgae and cyanobacteria-a review on current methodologies. Applied Sciences (Switzerland). 2021;**11**(11):1-20. DOI: 10.3390/app11115187

[6] Komárek J, Johansen JR. Filamentous cyanobacteria. In: Freshwater Algae of North America: Ecology and Classification. San Diego, CA: Elsevier Inc.; 2015. pp. 135-235. DOI: 10.1016/B978-0-12-385876-4.00004-9

[7] Allaf MM, Peerhossaini H. Cyanobacteria: Model microorganisms and beyond. Microorganisms. 2022;**10**(4):1-23. DOI: 10.3390/microorganisms10040696

[8] Brahamsha B, Bhaya D. Motility in unicellular and filamentous cyanobacteria. In: The Cell Biology of Cyanobacteria. Norfolk, UK: Caister Academic Press; 2014. pp. 233-262

[9] Castenholz RW. General characteristics of the cyanobacteria. In: Bergey's Manual of Systematics of Archaea and Bacteria. New Jersey: Wiley; 2015. pp. 1-23. DOI: 10.1002/9781118960608.cbm00019

[10] Herrero A, Stavans J, Flores E. The multicellular nature of filamentous heterocyst-forming cyanobacteria. FEMS Microbiology Reviews. 2016;**40**(6):831-854. DOI: 10.1093/femsre/fuw029

[11] Garcia-Pichel F, Zehr JP, Bhattacharya D, Pakrasi HB. What's in a name? The case of cyanobacteria. Journal of Phycology. 2020;**56**(1):1-5. DOI: 10.1111/jpy.12934

[12] Do Nascimento Junior JR, Zevallos Torres LA, Medeiros ABP, Woiciechowski AL, Martinez-Burgos WJ, Soccol CR. Enhancement of biohydrogen production in industrial wastewaters with vinasse pond consortium using lignin-mediated iron nanoparticles. International Journal of Hydrogen Energy. 2021;**46**(54):27431-27443. DOI: 10.1016/j.ijhydene.2021.06.009

[13] Martinez-Burgos WJ, Junior JR, et al. Biohydrogen production from agro-industrial wastes using *Clostridium beijerinckii* and isolated bacteria as inoculum. BioEnergy Research. 2021;**15**(1):18. DOI: 10.1007/s12155-021-10358-1

[14] Severo IA, Siqueira SF, Deprá MC, Maroneze MM, Zepka LQ, Jacbo-Lopes E. Biodiesel facilities: What can we address to make biorefineries commercially competitive? Renewable and Sustainable Energy Reviews. 2019;**112**:686-705. DOI: 10.1016/j.rser.2019.06.020

[15] Cordeiro RS, Vaz ICD, Magalhães SMS, Barbosa FAR. Effects of nutritional conditions on lipid production by cyanobacteria. Anais Da Academia Brasileira de Ciencias. 2021;**89**(3):2021-2031. DOI: 10.1590/0001-3765201720150707

[16] Chowdury KH, Nahar N, Deb UK. The growth factors involved in microalgae cultivation for biofuel production: A review. Computational Water, Energy, and Environmental Engineering. 2020;**09**(04):185-215. DOI: 10.4236/cweee.2020.94012

[17] Dexter J, Fu P. Metabolic engineering of cyanobacteria for ethanol production. Energy and Environmental Science. 2009;**2**(8):857-864. DOI: 10.1039/b811937f

[18] Liang F, Englund E, Lindberg P, Lindblad P. Engineered cyanobacteria with enhanced growth show increased ethanol production and higher biofuel to biomass ratio. Metabolic Engineering. 2018;**46**(November 2017):51-59. DOI: 10.1016/j.ymben.2018.02.006

[19] Bižić M, Klintzsch T, Ionescu D, Hindiyeh MY, Günthel M, Muro-Pastor AM, et al. Aquatic and terrestrial cyanobacteria produce methane. Science Advances. 2020;**6**(3):1-9. DOI: 10.1126/sciadv.aax5343

[20] Huang R, McGrath SP, Hirsch PR, Clark IM, Storkey J, Wu L, et al. Plant–microbe networks in soil are weakened by century-long use of inorganic fertilizers. Microbial Biotechnology. 2019;**12**(6):1464-1475. DOI: 10.1111/1751-7915.13487

[21] Joshi H, Shourie A, Singh A. Cyanobacteria as a source of biofertilizers for sustainable agriculture. Advances in Cyanobacterial Biology. 2020;**22**:385-396. DOI: 10.1016/B978-0-12-819311-2.00025-5

[22] Paredes I, Otero N, Soler A, Green AJ, Soto DX. Agricultural and urban delivered nitrate pollution input to Mediterranean temporary freshwaters. Agriculture, Ecosystems and Environment. 2020;**294**:106859. DOI: 10.1016/j.agee.2020.106859

[23] Rashid A, Mir MR, Hakeem KR. Biofertilizer use for sustainable agricultural production. In: Plant, Soil and Microbes. Switzerland: Springer Cham; 2016

[24] Song T, Mårtensson L, Eriksson T, Zheng W, Rasmussen U. Biodiversity and seasonal variation of the cyanobacterial assemblage in a rice paddy field in Fujian, China. FEMS Microbiology Ecology. 2005a;**54**(1):131-140. DOI: 10.1016/j.femsec.2005.03.008

[25] Rodríguez A, Stella A, Storni M, Zulpa G, Zaccaro M. Effects of cyanobacterial extracellular products and gibberellic acid on salinity tolerance in *Oryza sativa* L. Saline Systems. 2006;**2**(1):1-4. DOI: 10.1186/1746-1448-2-7

[26] Saadatnia H, Riahi H. Cyanobacteria from paddy fields in Iran as a biofertilizer in rice plants. Plant, Soil and Environment. 2009;**55**(5):207-212. DOI: 10.17221/384-pse

[27] Severo IA, de Lira GS, Ambati RR, Gokare RA, Vargas JVC, Ordonez J, et al. Disruptive potential of microalgae proteins: Shaping the future of the food industry. Future Foods. 2024;**9**:100318. DOI: 10.1016/j.fufo.2024.100318

[28] Ferrazzano GF, Papa C, Pollio A, Ingenito A, Sangianantoni G, Cantile T. Cyanobacteria and microalgae as sources of functional foods to improve human

general and oral health. Molecules. 2020;**25**(21):1-17. DOI: 10.3390/molecules25215164

[29] Ahmed E. Antimicrobial activity of microalgal extracts isolated from Baharia Oasis, Egypt. Environmental Science, Medicine, Biology. 2016;**5**:33-41

[30] Vijayakumar S, Menakha M. Pharmaceutical applications of cyanobacteria: A review. Journal of Acute Medicine. 2015;**5**:15-23

[31] Naga Pavan Kumar B, Mahaboobi S, Satyam S. Cyanobacteria: A potential natural source for drug discovery and bioremediation. Journal of Industrial Pollution Control. 2016;**32**(2):508-517

[32] Severo IA, Dias RR, do Nascimento, T.C., et al. Microalgae-derived polysaccharides: Potential building blocks for biomedical applications. World Journal of Microbiology and Biotechnology. 2022;**38**:150. DOI: 10.1007/s11274-022-03342-0

[33] Sánchez-Baracaldo P, Bianchini G, Wilson JD, Knoll AH. Cyanobacteria and biogeochemical cycles through Earth history. Trends in Microbiology. 2022;**30**(2):143-157. DOI: 10.1016/j.tim.2021.05.008

[34] Chakdar H, Thapa S, Srivastava A, Shukla P. Genomic and proteomic insights into the heavy metal bioremediation by cyanobacteria. Journal of Hazardous Materials. 2022;**424**:127609. DOI: 10.1016/j.jhazmat.2021.127609

[35] Potnis AA, Raghavan PS, Rajaram H. Overview on cyanobacterial exopolysaccharides and biofilms: Role in bioremediation. Reviews in Environmental Science and Biotechnology. 2021;**20**(3):781-794. DOI: 10.1007/s11157-021-09586-w

[36] Fokina AI, Ogorodnikova SY, DomrachevaLI,LyalinaEI,GornostaevaEA, Ashikhmina TY, et al. Cyanobacteria as test organisms and biosorbents. Eurasian Soil Science. 2017;**50**(1):70-77. DOI: 10.1134/S106422931611003X

Chapter 2

Advances in Spirulina Cultivation: Techniques, Challenges, and Applications

Maja Berden Zrimec, Eleonora Sforza, Leonardo Pattaro, Davide Carecci, Elena Ficara, Antonio Idà, Narcís Ferrer-Ledo, Stefano Canziani, Silvio Mangini, Borut Lazar, Sophia Papadaki, Giorgos Markou, Ioannis Tzovenis and Robert Reinhardt

Abstract

Spirulina is a microalga recognized for its nutritional benefits and its potential in sustainable food production. Existing large-scale cultivation produces spirulina of very different quality, taste, and odor. The reason lies in various approaches to the production, which range from the low-technology simple systems to high-end high-quality production for more demanding consumer market. In this chapter, we present challenges and possible solutions to ensure production of high-grade spirulina. We describe the design and crucial demands that have to be assured in the production system. The quality and productivity can be further increased by applying a bioprocess engineering approach based on modeling of the cultivation. Thermal modeling is also presented as an approach to optimize cultivation in the greenhouse systems. A spirulina production in Italy is showcased to pinpoint challenges of spirulina production in Europe. We conclude with an extensive study of regulatory framework for the spirulina production that must be taken into account for the successful algae production.

Keywords: spirulina, large-scale production, food, high-grade quality, algae production

1. Introduction

The commercial production of spirulina is well-established worldwide. In fact, spirulina is the most extensively cultivated microalga in Europe with over 200 facilities generating almost 150 tons of dry biomass annually [1]. Worldwide production in 2019 was evaluated by FAO as 56,208 tons [2]. The global spirulina market size reached € 533 million in 2023. Looking forward, IMARC Group expects the market to reach €1189.6 million by 2032, exhibiting a growth rate (CAGR) of 9.33% during 2024–2032 [3].

IntechOpen

Nevertheless, its potential in Europe remains largely untapped as its cultivation typically takes place in tropical or semitropical regions favorable for spirulina growth.

Spirulina is a common name for commercial strains of cyanobacteria species *Arthrospira platensis* and *A. maxima*, also known by the old genus name *Spirulina* or recently even *Limnospira* (phylum Cyanobacteria) [4, 5]. While taxonomists name species according to their genetic relations as new data are discovered, technologists prefer to use common names that remain stable over time as consistency is needed in practical applications. Spirulina has long, thin filaments that are typically arranged in a spiral or helical shape, which is its distinctive feature (**Figure 1**). The helices can be tight or loose, depending on the environmental conditions. The cells are cylindrical and quite small, usually about 2 to 8 μm in diameter, but filaments can be up to several hundred μm long. The intense blue-green color of spirulina is due to the presence of chlorophyll and phycocyanin.

Spirulina has high intraspecies diversity, independent of phylogenetic affiliations or geographical locations, indicating significant physiological and metabolic plasticity [5]. This genetic variation underpins its physiological and metabolic flexibility, essential for its wide range of applications.

Spirulina thrives in alkaline environment (pH range 9.5–11) and prefers moderate to relatively high temperatures. Optimal growth conditions reported for spirulina are in the range of 300–500 μmol photons m^{-2} s^{-1} and 25–35°C [6, 7]. However, it can also tolerate a wide range of conditions, which contributes to its widespread distribution.

Cultivated worldwide, spirulina is used as a dietary supplement or whole food ingredient. It is very rich in proteins and antioxidant compounds. Spirulina is used for the extraction of pigments such as phycocyanin, a blue photosynthetic pigment which is used in health, cosmetics, and food applications [1]. It is also used as a feed supplement in the aquaculture, aquarium, and poultry industries. Spirulina contains numerous essential nutrients, like B vitamins (thiamine, riboflavin, and niacin), and dietary minerals, such as iron and manganese [8].

The goal of this study was to address the challenges associated with large-scale spirulina cultivation and to provide guidance on producing high-grade biomass for discerning markets. Our approach utilized bioprocess engineering to achieve high-quality cultivation through enhanced environmental control in greenhouses, improved design and operations, and optimized culturing procedures. The study concludes with a detailed examination of the regulatory frameworks essential for successful spirulina production.

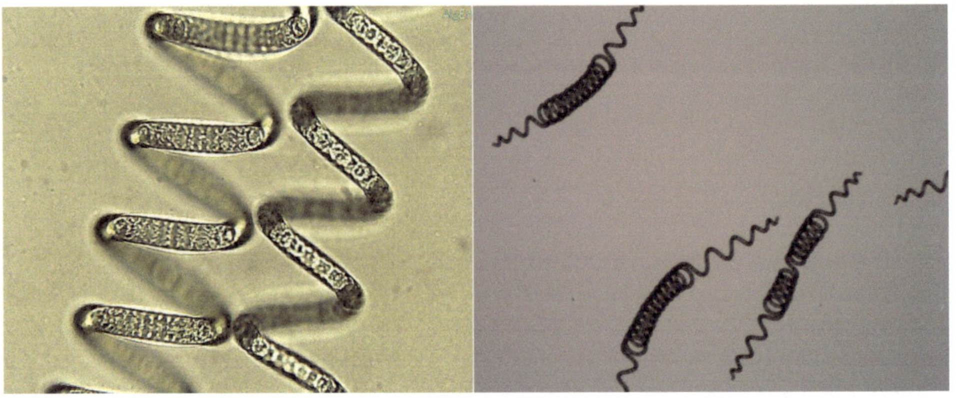

Figure 1.
Spirulina with its distinctive spiral shape.

2. Cultivation approaches, challenges, and solutions for high-grade production

Flourishing in extreme conditions characterized by high pH levels and temperatures, spirulina cultures can be very resistant to contamination. Consequently, most of the producers prefer open ponds (83% of companies in EU [1]) due to their significantly lower cost compared to photobioreactors. Pond systems consist of a raceway pond where water is mixed with a paddlewheel (**Figure 2**). They can be installed outdoors, meaning they are open to the environment, utilizing natural sunlight for algae growth, or can be housed in greenhouses for better control of the environmental conditions and prevention of infections. There are several general approaches to cultivation of spirulina for food, including (i) low technology simple systems, (ii) industrial style production in open ponds for middle quality and high-volume biomass, (iii) high-end high-quality system addressing the new-age consumer market. Each approach represents different biomass safety and quality. This chapter will present approaches for high-grade spirulina production.

2.1 Main challenges

Several factors lower the quality of current spirulina production. Open ponds offer no defense against contamination from dirt, insects, or animal remains, exposing spirulina to various environmental elements. The only form of protection employed is the regulation of pH levels to deter foreign species.

Spirulina's quality is sometimes criticized due to concerns over contaminants. Heavy metals, such as arsenic, lead, and mercury, can be absorbed by spirulina from the environment, especially when grown in open ponds subjected to pollution.

Bacterial contamination and the presence of cyanotoxins are also of concern, as spirulina is often cultivated in environments conducive to the proliferation of various microorganisms, including harmful bacteria and cyanobacteria.

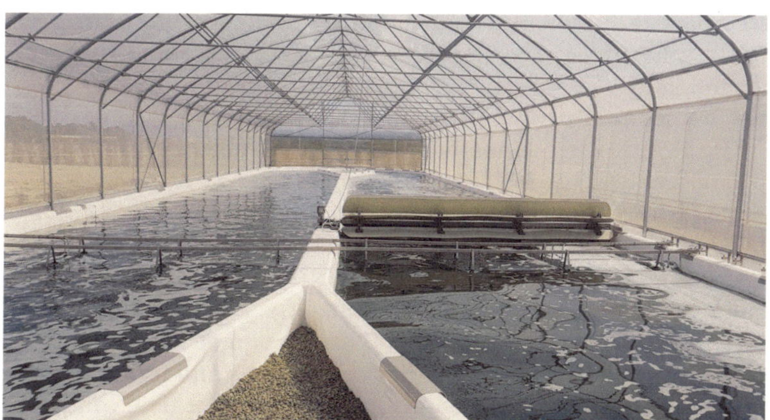

Figure 2.
Spirulina production in raceway pond in a greenhouse (Grosseto, Italy; Source: Algen archive).

Another point of criticism is the presence of polycyclic aromatic hydrocarbons (PAHs), which can form during the high-temperature drying process of spirulina. PAHs are known to be carcinogenic, and their presence in food products is highly regulated.

In the process of harvesting, media washing is done to purify the spirulina, but this step can also remove beneficial extracellular ingredients. Furthermore, the focus of current production is on optimizing the growth rate to increase the yield, rather than enhancing the quality of the spirulina.

The design, safety, and quality aspects of large-scale spirulina cultivation is thus critical for ensuring a successful operation. The design focuses on creating a controlled environment that maximizes spirulina growth while minimizing contamination risks (**Figure 2**). Safety measures include maintaining high cleanliness standards to ensure the product is free from contaminants like heavy metals and bacteria. Quality is achieved through a combination of design decisions such as closed ponds, uniform mixing, and low-temperature processing. These components work together to produce high-grade spirulina that is safe, of high quality, and produced efficiently on a large scale.

2.2 Pond systems for high-quality spirulina cultivation

High-grade spirulina cultivation should be meticulously undertaken with carefully designed ponds. Ponds need to be either covered or fully enclosed, preferably with insect nets, to shield spirulina from external contaminants such as dust, insects, and bird droppings. The pond bottom should be constructed with high-quality materials that prevent the growth of undesirable bacteria and facilitate easy cleaning.

The shape of the pond should be designed to prevent the formation of eddies, thus ensuring uniform spirulina growth and reducing energy consumption. The flow within the pond must be evenly distributed, a task accomplished by installing vanes or deflectors that spread the flow across the entire length of the pond, ensuring all parts receive equal amounts of nutrients and light. The inclusion of slanted walls can enhance wave behavior, helping to prevent stagnation and promote uniform cultivation conditions.

Regular cleaning should be conducted to maintain a pristine environment for the spirulina. Temperature regulation is critical; in hotter climates, forced air evaporation cooling systems are recommended to maintain an optimal growth temperature, while in cooler climates, heating can be effectively managed with immersed heat exchangers to avoid contamination.

Moreover, to prevent oxygen build-up, which can stress spirulina cells, a stripping sump should be included in the pond design. This will ensure that oxygen levels are balanced, promoting healthy growth and preventing oxidative damage.

Adhering to these design principles should ensure the cultivation of high-grade spirulina, yielding a product that is both safe and nutritionally rich for the consumer market (**Figure 3**).

The piping system is essential for maintaining the integrity and cleanliness of the culture environment in spirulina cultivation. Key design decisions include rigorous post-use washing of all media pipes to remove remnants and prevent contamination, strategic valve placement near the ponds for better nutrient flow control and reduced contamination risk, and the implementation of an agitation system to keep growth media in motion, addressing stagnant media issues, maintaining media quality, and preventing pipe blockages.

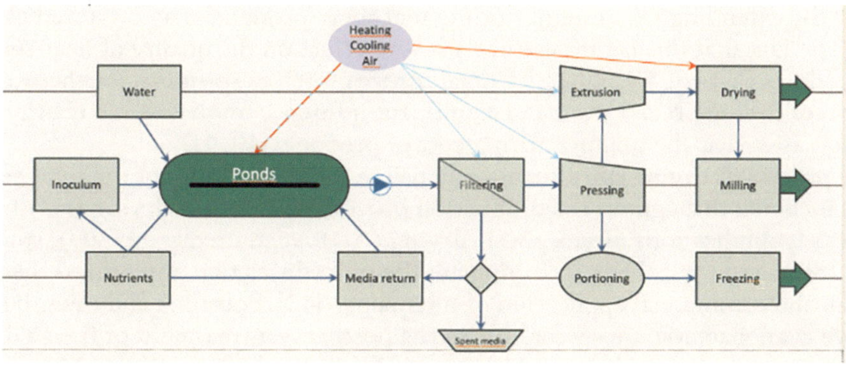

Figure 3.
Top-level schematic illustrates the comprehensive workflow for spirulina production, from inoculum and nutrient preparation through various processing stages like filtering, pressing, drying, freezing, milling, and extrusion. This schematic underscores the importance of a systematic approach to spirulina cultivation and processing, highlighting the necessity of careful planning in each stage to ensure the highest quality of the final product. The inclusion of media return and spent media management also indicates the sustainability considerations inherent in the production design.

Comprehensive spirulina cultivation strategy is thus based on maintaining a clean and controlled environment to ensure high-quality production. The pH level is maintained above 10.5 to reduce growth rate slightly (in comparison to pH 9.5) but increase safety, with meticulous monitoring and adjustments using NaOH or KOH (depends on the further use of spent media for fertigation). Sufficient cleanliness is achieved with covered ponds, stringent entry protocols, and rigorous pest control measures. The system is designed to minimize stagnant culture areas and ensure all water used is sterilized (UVC at 5.3 Wh/m^3), filtered, and deionized to remove most of the cations like, Ca and Mg, to prevent precipitation and white or brown flakes in biomass. Continuous Cleaning-In-Place (CIP) procedures, including post-use washes (bleach daily), washing paddlewheels and pond edges, brushing the pond lining, and regular sanitation, are enforced. The operational protocols include microscopic examinations, toxin checks, and genetic monitoring to ensure spirulina's health and safety.

2.3 Processing of biomass

Spirulina processing occurs in a controlled clean room environment to prevent contamination. For the filtering process in high-grade spirulina production, it is essential to conduct filtering at low temperatures, specifically 5–10°C, to minimize the risk of biomass degradation. The system avoids the use of water chilling and/or heat exchangers to prevent the risk of stalled biomass, ensuring the integrity of the spirulina during the filtration process. Implementing these measures within a clean room environment further ensures the purity and quality of the spirulina, safeguarding it from potential contaminants.

The process of dehydration is an essential practice for the preservation of food products over an extended length of time. In addition to reducing the development of germs, it also slows down other processes that cause deterioration. Agricultural goods undergo negative structural, textural, and biochemical changes as a result of traditional drying procedures, which leads to a significant reduction in the sensory qualities and nutritional value of the products [9]. However, drying is still an effective method for extending the amount of time that these products may be stored effectively. The fact that this is the case has a severe effect on the quality of heat-sensitive food products that have a high nutritional content, such as spirulina. Furthermore, the selection of drying procedures has a significant influence on the overall energy consumption as well as the manufacturing cost of products [10, 11].

The process of drying spirulina is responsible for around 30% of the total expenditures incurred throughout the production process [12]. Freeze drying (FD) (also known as lyophilization), atmospheric drying (AD), vacuum drying (VD), spray drying (SD), and typical hot air drying are the procedures that are utilized the most often for the commercial application of microalgae [12]. Spirulina and other heat-sensitive cyanobacteria are susceptible to the postharvest treatment of freeze drying, which is commonly considered to be a successful method. According to Marques and Freire [13] and Oliveira *et al.* [14], this technique reduces several changes that occur to the nutritional, sensory, and physicochemical qualities of the components, which ultimately results in lyophilized products that are very similar to fresh biomass. However, in comparison to other popular drying processes, such as normal air drying, which is a more cost-effective method [15], freeze drying requires a significant amount of additional energy consumption as well as expensive equipment. On the other hand, vacuum drying provides a number of significant advantages in comparison to the conventional atmospheric drying method. These advantages include a quicker drying rate and a processing environment with lower levels of oxygen and other gases. According to Šumić *et al.* [16] and Wu *et al.* [9], these characteristics offer a significant contribution to the preservation of the quality and nutritional content of the dehydrated goods while simultaneously decreasing the expenditures that are connected with them. The spray drying process results in a high operating temperature of about 180°C, which has a detrimental impact on the quality of the dried spirulina microalga biomass. Agustini *et al.*'s work [17] suggests this is due to the fact that the heat-sensitive and essential components experience high levels of deterioration at temperatures of this magnitude.

The drying process is critical for preserving the nutritional quality of spirulina. Drying microalgal biomass is an essential process that enables the storage, processing, and transportation of the raw material. However, drying is a highly energy-intensive process that significantly impacts the ultimate structural and nutritional properties of the end product. According to Papadaki *et al.* [18], the wet spirulina biomass exhibits the maximum concentration of pigments and antioxidant activity, but a notable decline in bioactivity is found in the dry samples. Accelerated solar drying (ASD) demonstrated superior performance in the recovery of phycocyanin, whereas vacuum drying (VD) yielded a greater quantity of total carotenoids. In addition, the ASD process exhibited a greater environmental imprint across all categories, whereas the cultivation and harvesting phase of VD prior to drying demonstrated an exceptionally high carbon and energy footprint. The biomass acquired following VD exhibited a low concentration of phycocyanin, necessitating an increased feedstock quantity to yield the 1 kg of phycocyanin designated as the functional unit in the life cycle assessment. The environmental impact of phycocyanin production will be considerably diminished when one considers that the environmental footprint of microalgae production can be attributed to other products as well, including total carotenoids, chlorophylls, antioxidant compounds, and the polysaccharides of the microalgae themselves.

The decision to avoid spray dryers, which can cause high-temperature loss of essential spirulina properties (ESP), is a significant one. Instead, the production process utilizes a warm air dryer operating at 40–45°C, ensuring quick drying within 2–

3 hours. This method, combined with the use of a belt with non-sticking mesh or trays, effectively maintains spirulina's nutritional integrity. The air used in the process is dehumidified (chilled to 5°C) before being warmed to 40–45°C, with a multistage belt dryer or stacked net used to conserve space. This process also takes place in a clean room to ensure the highest quality and purity of the final product.

Stramarkou *et al*. [19] compared four methods of drying *Spirulina platensis*—atmospheric, freeze, vacuum, and accelerated solar—and found that the vacuum drying was the most effective in recovering the carotenoid content and to accomplish the quickest reduction in moisture content. Although atmospheric drying is considered an optimal technique for the preservation of phycocyanin and phenolic compounds, its protracted dehydration period renders it unsuitable for industrial implementation. Although freeze drying proved to be the most effective method for recovering β-carotene, it entails significant fixed and operating expenses. Biomass desiccated *via* solar acceleration exhibited the greatest antioxidant activity, despite the fact that a substantial degradation of the diverse bioactive compounds under investigation took place.

Packing the spirulina soon after drying and ensuring it is hermetically sealed are crucial steps for preserving its quality. The storage of the packaged product occurs in a clean area—grade 2, further emphasizing the importance of maintaining a contaminant-free environment. For fresh spirulina, packing takes place in a filter room, ensuring that the freshness and nutritional value are locked in immediately after processing.

To ensure the purity of the air within the production facility, the inlet air undergoes two-stage filtration to remove dust and microparticles, including a coarse filter followed by a HEPA filter that guarantees 99.99% filtration efficacy. The air is chilled and dehumidified to specific conditions (10°C and 9 g H2O/m^3 for the filter room; warmed to 40°C and RH 18% for the dryer room) to support the spirulina processing requirements. Moreover, air handling includes overpressure in clean areas and specific flow rates, alongside small side passes of chilled and warm air for different rooms, to maintain optimal environmental conditions for spirulina processing.

3. Optimizing cultivation: modeling

Besides the technological constraints, attention should also be paid to the effect of operating variables on the biomass viability and productivity. The selection of the proper cultivation method is pivotal for a successful production, with harvested biomass concentration and productivity standing as key parameters for such a target. A first discussion should be focused on the cultivation mode. Batch cultivation in open raceways ponds represents one of the most widespread techniques within the industrial microalgae framework, with the major advantages of reduced capital and installation costs [20]. However, such strategy does not allow to maintain stable harvested biomass concentrations and productivities, with the self-shading phenomenon and nutrient variability acting as the first causes in prolonged cultivations like these [21]. The adoption of continuous approaches should be considered in order to stabilize biomass productivity and composition: in fact, once the residence time (the ratio between the reactor volume and the inlet flow rate) is set, a steady state is naturally established, with an obtained biomass productivity and quality constant over time [22]. Continuous operation can be done by stabilizing the inlet flow rate to keep constant the residence time (chemostat) or by selecting a set point of biomass concentration in the reactor, which is monitored by a turbidimeter and kept constant with a flow rate control, thus changing the residence time (turbidostat). However, due to technological limitations in the downstream and resulting increased initial investments for control devices, continuous operation is not yet exploited, not even at the pilot scale [23]. For these reasons, the semicontinuous cultivation mode is the most consolidated one at larger scale so far, based on removal of a certain amount of culture volume at discrete intervals, to partially harvest the biomass and replete nutrient supply. Semicontinuous operation mode at larger scale could however be improved by the knowledge acquired by lab continuous experience. As demonstrated before, the main operative condition affecting algal productivity and composition is the residence time. This applies also to semicontinuous cultivation, where the frequency and amount of harvested volume corresponds to an average residence time, according to Eq. (1):

$$\tau_{av} = \frac{volume\ of\ the\ reactor}{volume\ removed/time} \tag{1}$$

Thus, also in semicontinuous practice, the residence time should be properly adjusted to adjust biomass composition and improve productivity. Both the chemostat and turbidostat mode rationales can be applied with this perspective. The feasibility of spirulina cultivation under an optimized semicontinuous rationale was proved in the work of Pastore *et al.* [24], where *A. platensis* growth performances were tested on a 3.4 m^3 pilot-scale PBR adjusting the harvesting frequency to optimize harvested biomass concentration as well as inner composition, with particular focus on protein accumulation. Thus, the investigation of the effect of operating variable at lab scale is still a powerful source of information that can be translated into good practices at larger scale, if coupled with modeling and process simulation approaches. Research at laboratory scale can be carried out to optimize the overall process performances by acting on the operating conditions. One of the aspects of interest is the effect of uncoupling the solid retention time (SRT) and the hydraulic retention time (HRT), which represents a good strategy in this perspective, as demonstrated by Barbera *et al.* [25]. Indeed, this study shows the former as the key parameter for controlling the biomass concentration within the reactor, to achieve a proper light attenuation profile according to the incident light, and thus working at the compensation point, which is the optimal one to increase the photosynthetic efficiency. On the other hand, this biomass concentration is often low, with strong impact on the water to be supplied. Thus, the process configuration for SRT < HRT is the most interesting one, as it allows to recycle the culture medium when the maximization of biomass production is the aim of the system. In this way, it is possible to meet both process performances and sustainability; the reduction of the SRT allows to stay as close as possible to the optimum value of specific light supply rate, thus benefiting in terms of biomass productivity, while the increase of the HRT minimizes the input of water and nutrients to the process, as this configuration accounts for at least a partial medium recycling. From an operational perspective, the recovery of the medium introduces a third variable to the process, namely, the recycling ratio (R); defined as the proportion between the recycled flow rate and the integrating hold up one, it can be accordingly retrieved from the selected recovered medium percentage.

The necessity of finding the optimal process operative conditions can benefit from mathematical models: being able to reduce the actual processes in the form of mathematical equations allows to produce virtual cultivation forecasts, adjustable on the selected operating conditions, namely, the inputs given to the models themselves. Moreover, the development of mathematical models covers an important role in the overall bioprocesses design path, as it represents an essential step for scaling up operations. For a successful buildout, along with the selection of the independent material balances of the process, the correct definition of biomass kinetics must be pursued; indeed, a compromise between accuracy and simplicity must be found, usually achieved by picking the most important factors affecting such phenomenon. In mathematical terms, the most used models account for the effects of temperature, light, and nutrients availability, which are included in specifically tailored corrective factors, to reduce the species maximum specific rate of growth μ_{max} as in Eq. (2):

$$R_X = \mu C_X = \left[\mu_{max}\, \varphi(T) f(I) f(C,N,P) - \mu_{e,max}\, f_{maint}(I)\right] C_X \tag{2}$$

To account for the effect of operating temperature $\varphi(T)$, one of the most consolidated functions is the cardinal temperature model with inflection [26], in which the operating value is compared with the maximum T_{max}, minimum T_{min} and optimum T_{opt} species temperatures, as reported in Eq. (3).

$$\varphi(T) = \frac{(T - T_{max})(T - T_{min})^2}{\left(T_{opt} - T_{min}\right)\left[\left(T_{opt} - T_{min}\right)\left(T - T_{opt}\right) - \left(T_{opt} - T_{max}\right)\left(T_{opt} + T_{min} - 2T\right)\right]} \tag{3}$$

Concerning the light effect, several models are available [27, 28], but all should include the self-shading effect due to light absorption by biomass: this phenomenon produces an exponentially decreasing trend for light availability along the reactor depth coordinate z, commonly described by the Lambert-Beer law. Here, we present, as an example, the modified Haldane model representing the $f(I)$ in Eq. (4) [12]:

$$f(I) = \frac{1}{L}\int_0^L \frac{I(z)}{I(z) + K_I\left(\frac{I(z)}{I_{opt}} - 1\right)^2}\; with\; I(z) = I_0 \exp(-k_a C_X z) \tag{4}$$

The nutrients availability dependency (mainly regarding carbon, nitrogen, and phosphorus), mostly described with respect to the most limited one, is usually modelled according to the Monod-like kinetics, reported in Eq. (5).

$$f(C_i) = \frac{C_i}{C_i + K_i} \tag{5}$$

Nevertheless, this model has a strong limitation, as it considers a fixed biomass on nutrient yield. For this reason, Droop model should be applied: indeed, by introducing the concept of limiting nutrient quota, namely, the amount stored within biomass, a more accurate description of microalgal uptake dynamics can be achieved [29].

Finally, the maintenance is added to the overall dynamics, with the maximum maintenance energy $\mu_{e,max}$ adjusted according to the light availability correction factor $f_{maint}(I)$ [30] in Eq. (6).

$$f_{maint}(I) = \frac{I_0}{I_0 + k_{I,m}} \tag{6}$$

Eq. (2), namely, the standard microbial kinetics, may be further modified by introducing other factors that can affect growth performances. For instance, the presence of some organic metabolites may inhibit cyanobacterial growth, which must be accordingly modeled. This is the case when a medium recycling configuration is adopted: indeed, inefficiencies in the harvesting system may lead to an ineffective separation of such compounds, which may then accumulate within the reaction environment. Specifically for *Spirulina* sp., the literature reports exopolysaccharides (EPS) and free fatty acids as the main contributors in relation to this. If, on one hand, the active inhibitory effect of fatty acids accumulation is taken for granted [31], the inhibition mechanism provided by EPS is still subjected to debate. For instance, some works sustain EPS active role in *Arthrospira platensis* growth inhibition, while others support a more indirect role, with EPS accumulation increasing medium viscosity and negatively affecting the subsequent biomass harvest: this may induce a reduction in filterability, leaving room for the buildup of inhibitory compounds within the reactor environment. For example, see [17, 32]. Regardless of the rationale, this confirms that EPS may be seen as the key component while accounting for a potential inhibition correction of biomass kinetics. These experimental findings could be beneficial in view of process optimization if accounted by proper modeling techniques, aimed at tracking the system performance while simultaneously keeping in mind such inhibitory phenomenon; this way, the degree of medium recovery up to a value such that the EPS concentration with the reactor environment can be kept under control.

4. Thermal modeling of raceway ponds for microalgae cultivation

4.1 The thermal model for the greenhouse-pond system (GPS)

Mathematical growth models have been recently developed to forecast the performances of microalgae cultivation systems and the consequent cost-effectiveness of temperature control schemes (see Section 3). Since temperature is a crucial input parameter, a proper thermal modeling is of great aid to the simulation accuracy. Although validated models for open air cultures are already available [33], thermal evaluations under greenhouse (GH) are less well-established; nevertheless, a GH is typically needed to limit exogenous contamination to produce medium to high-quality biomass.

The dynamic greenhouse thermal model taken as reference was developed by Li *et al*. and describes shallow ponds for aquaculture purposes covered by a GH equipped with two cover layers [34]. It is a mechanistic conceptual/gray-box model, based on the modeling of the major heat exchange mechanisms and heat/mass balances across each component of the system. The model (**Figure 4**) considers perfectly mixed/homogeneous layers in the three spatial dimensions as for the external air, the air between the covers (when present), the GH internal air, and the pond water so that model components include: (i) the external ambient air (e), (ii) the air between the external (c1) and internal (c2) covers of the inflated double-layer glazing, (iii) the greenhouse (GH) inside air (i), and (iv) the raceway water (w). The raceway is assumed to cover the whole GH floor, and the soil beneath the raceway (s) is assumed to have a vertical temperature gradient until the isothermal layer is reached, whose temperature is a Dirichlet boundary condition, and it is considered equal to the annual average value of the external air temperature profile.

The original model was adapted to raceway pond (RWP) configurations, and some extensions were made [35], such as: (i) the development of the model for single-cover

DOI: http://dx.doi.org/10.5772/intechopen.1005474

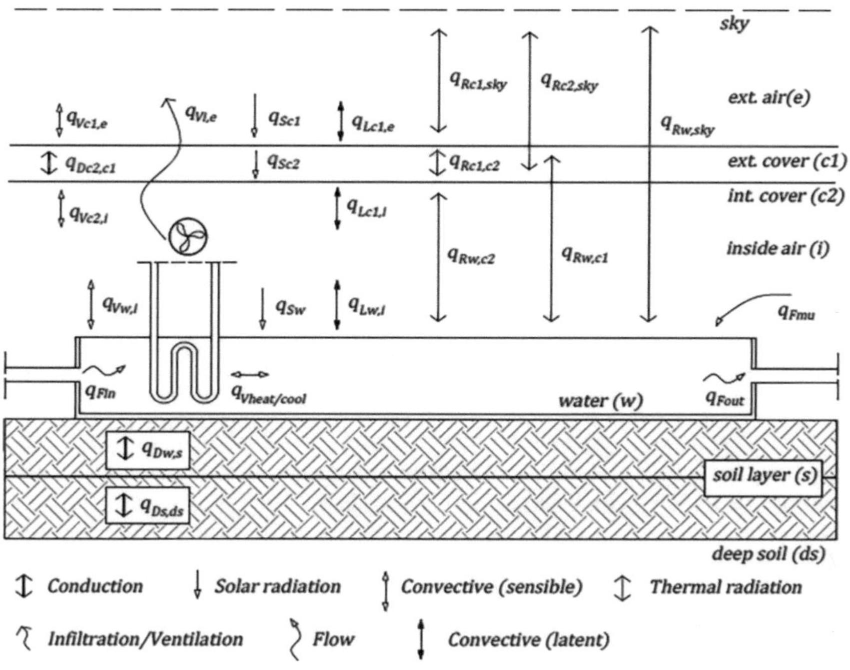

Figure 4.
Layers of the GHP system and heat fluxes for a double-cover GH.

(c) configuration, (ii) the presence of inflow/outflow and make-up water, (iii) the presence of RWP insulation, (iv) the possibility to apply temperature control strategies (water heating/cooling, mechanical ventilation), and (v) the impact of GH cover on the penetration of the photosynthetic active radiation (PAR).

4.1.1 Model structure

The overall differential algebraic equation (DAE) system is defined as in Eq. (7), where x are dynamic variables, z are algebraic variables, u are control inputs, θ are fixed parameters, d are external disturbances, and y are measurable outputs. Functions f and g are, without loss of generality, nonlinear (and in some cases $\in C^0$).

$$\begin{aligned} \dot{x} &= f(x,z,u,\theta,d) \\ 0 &= g(x,z,u,\theta,d) \\ y &= h(x,z,u,\theta,d) \end{aligned} \tag{7}$$

The state variables are three temperatures (T) of the interacting heat capacities and the water vapor content $e_{int,air}$ (kg m_{air}^{-3}) of the greenhouse internal air. The state variables interact with each other *via* heat fluxes Φ (W). The dynamic equations describe the energy balances for each uniform layer, that is:

$$CVdT/dt = Q(T_{in} - T) + \Phi(T,\theta,d) + u \tag{8}$$

where C (J m^{-3}°C^{-1}) is the volume-specific heat capacity and V (m^3) is the volume.

The first additive forcing term is related to the enthalpic contributions of inlet/outlet flows, where Q ($m^3\ s^{-1}$) is the flow rate, which are present only for the internal air and for the raceway pond (RWP) water layers. Water mass balance over the greenhouse internal air is used to calculate $e_{int,air}$, which is involved in the latent-convective heat exchange. The cover temperatures are algebraic variables (negligible heat capacity). With reference to **Figure 4**, the heat exchange mechanisms are:

- *Radiation qR*. As the covers have very high transmissivity, both covers and water pond are heated up by solar near-infrared radiation (NIR) during the day and cooled by far-infrared radiation (FIR) emission to the sky during the night. The thermal radiation properties of plastic covers vary with the amount of condensate covering them.

- *Sensible convection qV*. outside air convection is primarily impacted by greenhouse geometry and wind speed, whereas inner air convection is primarily influenced by temperature differences between layers. Heat exchange with external air is also considered *via* an infiltration rate *Ra* (h^{-1}). Although it varies with the inside-outside temperature difference and outside wind speed, the heat loss resulting from infiltration is generally small compared to the overall heat loss, and therefore, *Ra* was assumed to be constant.

- *Latent convection qL*. Heat exchange for water phase transition primarily depends on sensible convective heat transfer coefficient, Lewis number, and difference in water vapor concentration as driving force.

- *Conduction qD*. Conductive exchange is primarily present between the pond and the ground, and between the internal and external air.

The enthalpic contribution given by pond make-up water was also considered. The model has a time step resolution of 120 seconds.

The PAR ($\mu mol\ m^{-2}\ s^{-1}$) that reaches the pond surface is given by Eq. (9), that is:

$$PAR_w = 2.105\tau_{S,c}^2(1 - \rho_{S,w})I_0 \tag{9}$$

where 2.105 is a conversion factor, $\tau_{S,c}$ is the transmissivity of each cover to solar radiation, $\rho_{S,w}$ is the reflectivity of the water surface, and I_0 is the outside global solar radiation ($W\ m^{-2}$).

4.1.2 Model parameters and input data

The GHP thermal model includes the following classes of parameters (θ): (i) empirical parameters subject to calibration, (ii) physical parameters (for example pond water, soil, and air thermal/optical properties), (iii) empirical parameters from literature correlations (for example sky/external air temperatures correlation), and (iv) input design parameters (for example hydraulic retention time (HRT), pond liquid height, GH geometry, and cover material properties).

As a matter of fact, compromise between model complexity, computational time, and modeling effort was made so that the model contains both conceptual correlations and 6 empirical parameters subject to case-specific calibration; these are: (i) the infiltration rate *(Ra)*, (ii) the thickness of the non-isothermal soil layer (*Ls*), (iii) the convection regime between the cover layers (k_1 multiplier coefficient of $qD_{c1,c2}$—in case of a double cover), (iv) the reflection contributions to solar irradiance from the surroundings to the greenhouse external layer (k_2 multiplier coefficient of qS_c), (v) the convective heat transfer coefficient between water and internal air (k_3 multiplier coefficient of $hV_{w,i}$), and (vi) the convective heat transfer coefficient between internal air and internal cover (k_4 multiplier coefficient of $hV_{i,c2}$).

The inputs to the GPS model are process design parameters and weather data. Hourly weather data are required for: (i) external air temperature (*Te*), (ii) global solar irradiance at ground level (I_0), (iii) external air relative humidity (*RHe*), and (iv) external air wind velocity (*ue*).

4.1.3 Temperature control

The GPS model was integrated with a pond water temperature feedback control scheme (es. multiple input single output (MISO) proportional-integral-derivative (PID) control) for the estimation of: (i) the heating/cooling loads and peak powers from direct submerged heat-exchangers and (ii) the mechanical ventilation load and peak power. Mechanical ventilation was modeled with an additive term on *Ra*.

4.2 The integrated thermal and biological model

4.2.1 The opportunity of optimizing temperature regulation

Microalgae metabolism is particularly sensitive to temperature, and literature is rich in models that consider the effect of temperature on microalgae growth and respiration. An effective model that quantifies the temperature dependence of growth and respiration is the Cardinal Temperature Model with Inflection (CTMI) proposed by Rosso *et al.* [36] and reported in Eq. (3). It includes three parameters (the cardinal temperatures: Tmax, Topt, Tmin), which define the optimal working range for each microalgae strain [37]. In addition, temperature also plays a role in physiochemical equilibria, such as gas/liquid exchange, solubility, and dissociations that indirectly add impacts on metabolism.

When the GPS is integrated with biological or with biological and physical-chemical models, a comprehensive understanding of the algae biomass production facility can be run leading to a proper estimation of microalgae productivity and the consequent cost-effectiveness of thermal regulations. With calibrated GPS and biological growth models, the integrated assessment can be adapted to different climatic and biological conditions, allowing to improve the techno-economic analysis (TEA) and the consequent feasibility and scalability of microalgae cultivation. Indeed, an objective function that entails both the higher revenues and the higher costs from temperature regulation can be set for scenario analysis and optimization.

4.2.2 A case-study

An example is presented in Carecci [21], where the GPS is integrated to the comprehensive biological and physical-chemical ALBA model [38]. The simulations carried out with the ALBA model considers climate conditions as they are computed from the GPS model (water temperature (**Figure 5**), evaporation (m^3 day^{-1}), and light intensity (μmol m^{-2} s^{-1})). The case study considers a biorefinery located in

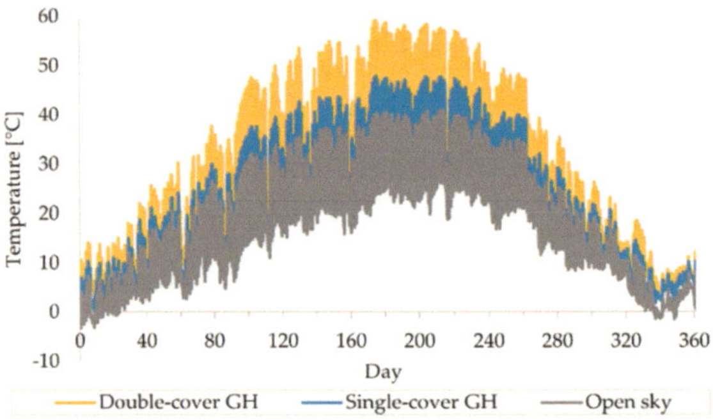

Figure 5.
Yearly RWP water temperature dynamics for open, single-covered, and double-covered GH configurations.

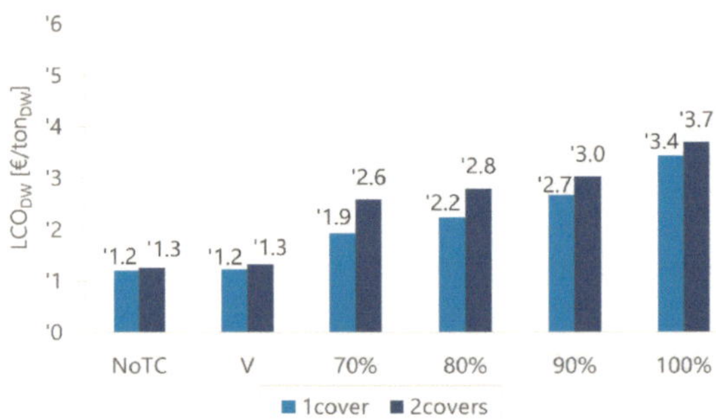

Figure 6.
Levelized costs of microalgae biomass production (LCO_DW) for different covering, control strategies, and set points scenario.

Lombardy (northern Italy) for the cultivation of a *Chlorella-Scenedesmus* consortia for biostimulant production on agrozootechnical liquid digestate. In that case study, different scenarios were evaluated considering different GH covering alternatives, water temperature set points, and temperature control strategies. The latter were selected by assuming different temperature ranges around the optimal value as suggested by the CTMI curve for that microalgae community, which would be allowed in the pond by the T-controller. The productivity computed from the ALBA model was combined with heating/cooling loads provided by the thermal control logic in a comprehensive economic framework, where levelized costs (**Figure 6**) and return of investments were evaluated. For the specific location and market conditions of the case study, the best design option was to implement a single-cover GH, regulated only by summer cooling *via* both mechanical ventilation and water-cooling. Similar simulations can be easily extended to spirulina production by adapting the biological model parameters to describe spirulina growth and respiration rates.

5. Upgrading the biomass quality

Besides the improvements on growth rates by applying different cultivation strategies (see sections above), biomass quality improvements in terms of its biochemical composition (proteins, carbohydrates, lipids, pigments, and mineral content) are also possible by controlling some of the cultivation parameters. The main parameters that can be considered for this purpose are light intensity and quality, time of harvest, nutrient availability, and salinity of the growth medium.

Light has not only an important role on the cell growth, but it influences the biochemical composition of the biomass. It is generally observed that at higher light intensities, the biosynthesis of carbohydrates is favored, while at lower intensities, the protein and pigment content (phycocyanin and chlorophyll) is higher. This is because at increased intensities (however below levels that cause photoinhibition), photosynthesis is improved and the photosynthate is directed towards the biosynthesis of carbon and energy storage compounds like glycogen, which then is utilized further as metabolic energy carrier for biosynthesis of other metabolites, or respiration. When artificial light is applied, the intensity could be optimized for growth and protein and phycocyanin productivity. However, light intensity is a parameter that could not be efficiently controlled in cultures grown with solar energy due to the high fluctuations during the day, where typically at midday, the highest intensities occur. At very high light intensities, photoinhibition typically takes place that decreases growth and negatively influences protein and phycocyanin content [39, 40]. In practice, where production is performed with solar light, shading of the cultures is of importance to avoid photoinhibition. Since the quality of the light influences the biochemical composition of spirulina, the shading of the cultures could be performed by using colored filters absorbing most of the incident light spectrum and allowing passing the desired ones. As was reported by Kilimtzidi *et al.* [41] in small-pilot open pond experiments, shading of spirulina with red filters improved the protein and phycocyanin content. Also, the harvesting time has an important effect on the biomass quality, since it has been observed that in the early morning, the percentage of the proteins and of essential amino acids is the highest [42, 43].

Spirulina is typically cultivated with growth media with relatively high bicarbonate concentrations and total salinities (as sodium ions) to avoid any significant contamination with other microalgae or cyanobacteria. The most common growth medium used for spirulina production is Zarrouk that contains around 5.5 g-Na+/L. It was found, however, that the protein content of spirulina was around 11% higher when lower total sodium ions (4 g-Na+/L) was used [44]. Nevertheless, despite that increasing salinity negatively affects protein content, the use of seawater to formulate the growth medium could be a strategy for replacing fresh water and the production of biomass with increased unsaturated lipids (Oleic acid, Cis-9 (C18:1), and Palmitoleic (C16:1)) [44, 45].

For improved protein content, another possible strategy is the addition of small amounts of glycerol (0.5–1.5 g/L) [46, 47]. However, this strategy could negatively impact the cultures since heterotrophic microorganisms can grow when organic carbon is applied, especially in open-pond facilities where no sterile or axenic conditions can be achieved.

Spirulina contains minerals such as iron, magnesium, calcium, zinc, and so on and could be a good source when used as a food or feed supplement. The increase of these minerals in the growth medium could lead to the increase of their content as it is having been demonstrated in several studies [48–50].

Despite that spirulina has been produced with the main target in its protein and phycocyanin content, novel products could be also developed focusing on other compounds like polysaccharides. In the study of Markou *et al.* [51] under phosphorus limitation, it was found that spirulina was significantly enriched in 1.3:1.6-β-Glucans, which are considered to have antitumor, anti-inflammation, and antiviral activities.

6. Showcase Algaria, Italy

To better understand the importance of operating variables on biomass productivity and quality, a case study is presented here, to highlight the aspects that should be carefully considered to fill the substantial gaps related to scaling up and industrialization efforts of spirulina cultivation. Practical experiences from operating commercial-scale facilities highlight deviations from standardized laboratory conditions, both in terms of duration and due to biotic and environmental factors. Long-term evaluations tailored to specific production needs are thus essential for assessing the industrial scaling up of this nascent industry, posing new challenges also to the lab scale studies. One of the primary challenges faced by raceway facilities is their exposure to ambient conditions, which introduces various variables such as dust, insects, and bird droppings.

While covering the raceway with a greenhouse and protecting it with mosquito netting could mitigate these issues, this solution may impact light availability. The transparent plastic cover of the greenhouse reduces light penetration, resulting in an average reduction of 50% throughout the year, with the maximum impact observed during the summer. Despite this drawback, the greenhouse environment offers effective thermal management, providing a potential solution to address low temperatures. With a temperature difference of around 10°C between inside and outside the greenhouse during daylight hours, this setup could significantly extend the productive seasons in temperate regions by 2 or 3 months. This extended growing period has the potential to enhance overall spirulina production and contribute to the sustainability and profitability of raceway facilities. However, during the wintertime in temperate zones, temperatures can still decrease below zero, so it may still be challenging to maintain temperatures above the critical threshold of around 15°C, necessary for maintenance, especially for thermophilic microorganisms like spirulina.

The fluctuations during the 24-hour cycle are also important as the physiological aspects of photosynthesis and respiration are primarily influenced by light and temperature. Relatively low temperatures coupled with high light intensities—a common occurrence during summer/spring mornings in temperate zones—can lead to photosystem damage. Vonshak and Richmond [52] demonstrated that photoinhibition can occur in outdoor cultures, resulting in up to a 30% loss of biomass production rate. This limitation emphasizes the importance of exploring alternative solutions or implementing supplementary heating systems to maintain consistent and optimal conditions for spirulina cultivation throughout the year.

Algaria company in Italy addresses this challenge by utilizing heat generated by a biogas plant for spirulina production. This approach effectively reduces the daily temperature variation by ±5°C and ensures that temperature never falls below 15°C [19]. As a result, spirulina production flourishes, with reported yields ranging from 6 $g/m^2 \ day^{-1}$ in winter to 16 $g/m^2 \ day^{-1}$ in summer. This demonstrates the potential of innovative solutions to enhance sustainability and profitability in raceway facilities, particularly in temperate climates.

As stressed in the previous sections, it is crucial to consider the production process and operations, as they significantly influence the final production output. Operational conditions interact in complex ways; that is why an integrated approach to analysis is necessary. While continuous operation is ideal, maintaining a fixed dilution rate or biomass composition at a large scale can be problematic due to climate fluctuations and operational difficulties. A common approach is the use of a semicontinuous mode, like chemostat or turbidostat as described in Section 2. Seasonal patterns, such as different growth rates and biomass concentrations in winter and summer, must be still considered. Challenges arise during periods of negative growth rates, often caused by factors such as low light availability and moderate temperatures, which increase organic matter consumption compared to production by photosynthesis. Key parameters affecting productivity, such as dilution rate and harvesting frequency, should be chosen based on physiological traits of the culture and the objectives of the production system. Misalignment between harvesting rates and growth rates can lead to culture collapse. Therefore, robust operational protocols and adaptive management strategies are essential to ensure consistent and efficient spirulina production in raceway facilities.

7. Regulatory framework for spirulina production

Regulatory and market demands must be thoroughly considered in the spirulina production. The spirulina market is characterized by a significant presence of small and medium-sized enterprises (SME) that produce and sell spirulina products directly to consumers (business-to-consumer approach). These companies are usually run by few people with a background in a specific sector that need to multitask in different work areas. When starting a spirulina business, it is fundamental to assess the regulatory framework affecting the different steps of the value chain. The regulatory framework can be regarded as a tree, where the different applications of spirulina products share a common root (permissions, waste management, etc.) and trunk (labor safety, equipment operation, etc.) (**Figure** 7). Spirulina regulation falls on the algae framework, and it is application is sometimes complex and demanding. This section aims to provide spirulina entrepreneurs with some insights and guidance through the regulatory framework surrounding spirulina production. Most importantly, algae production in Europe is costly partly explained using complex equipment (e.g., closed photobioreactors or systems inside greenhouses) and compliance with stringent laws and standards for safety and quality. The complex regulatory landscape in the European Union is the basis for high quality and certified production of spirulina. Nevertheless, the low production of high-quality spirulina in Europe in front of imports from countries with a larger production and older tradition often results in poor quality products filling the European market. Recognition by consumers of the connection between the regulatory framework and product quality should counterbalance the spirulina market in Europe.

First of all, it is necessary to define what spirulina is from a regulatory point of view in Europe. European Standards [53] and the EABA [54] integrate cyanobacteria, microalgae, macroalgae, and Labyrinthulomycetes in the same functional group (algae) due to their similarities in functional properties and derived products. Algae and algae products fall under the regulation of aquaculture products mainly due to their cultivation in aqueous medium [55, 56], despite sharing traits of a biotechnological process (microorganism) and agricultural process (autotrophic growth). It is therefore relevant to distinguish the end stage of the final product since it will determine the hygiene regulation that must be followed. On the one side, regulations referring to agriculture (primary production) will apply when the purpose is growing biomass and harvesting. On the other side, regulations referring to industrial production (transformation) will apply when the process includes concentration, extraction, purification, and packaging. Finally, Spirulina is nowadays mainly sold as a food supplement or nutraceutical, but in the last years, it has gained interest in different

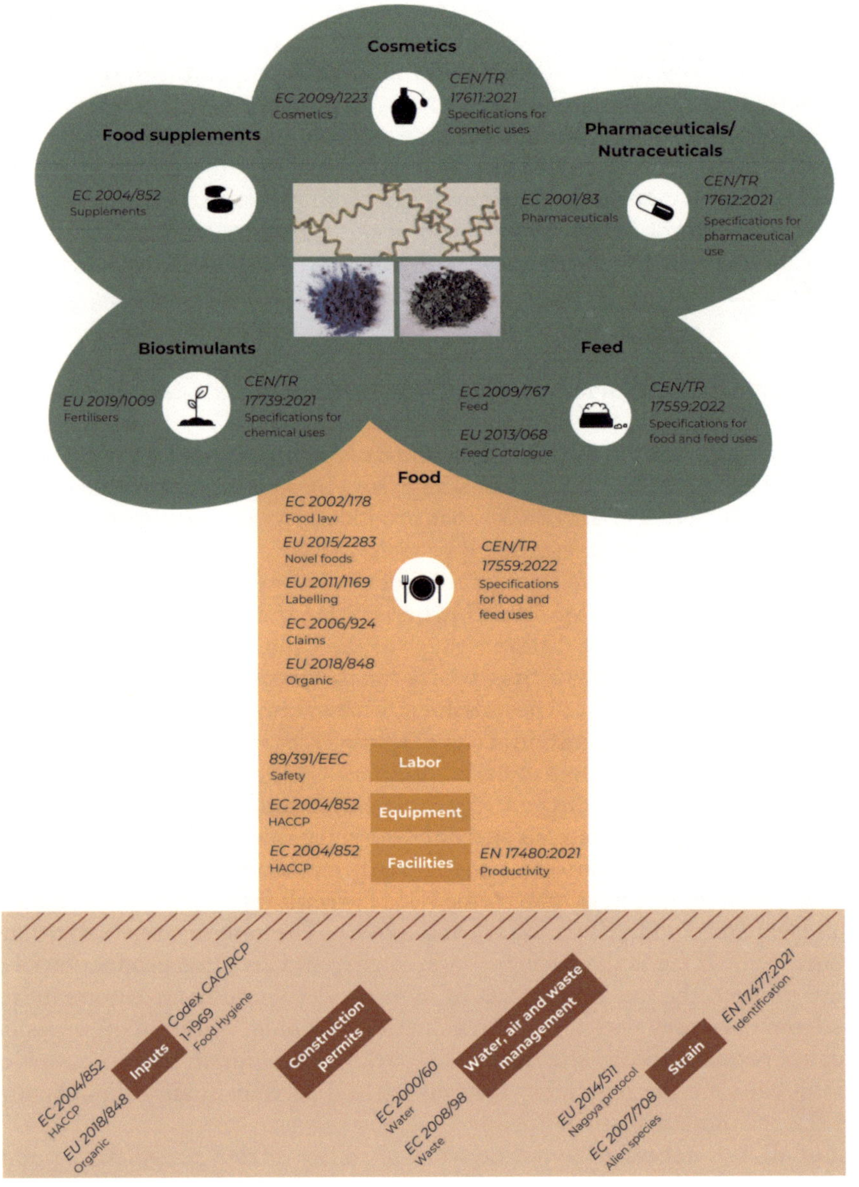

Figure 7.
Overview of the regulatory framework of spirulina products with special emphasis on the law and standards applying for products for the food sector. The scheme has a tree shape, distinguishing the most relevant laws for inputs, construction permits, waste management, and strain (roots); the laws/standards applying for labor, equipment, and facilities (trunk); and the laws/standards for the different applications of spirulina products (branches).

market sectors as a feed or biostimulant. Depending on the application of the final product, there will be a specific regulation to be applied. For instance, safety of food products is regulated by EC 178/2002 [57], but food supplements additionally require the compliance with directive 2002/46/EC [58]. The feed, cosmetic, and biostimulants sectors are regulated by the 2009/767/EC [59], the 2009/1223/EC [60], and the 2019/1009/EC [61], respectively. Regarding the nutraceutical or functional foods, there is not a specific regulation, and they may fall under those of pharmaceutical products (2001/83/EC [62], food for specific population groups (2013/609/EU [63]), or food supplements [33]. The following lines will focus on the use of spirulina for food and food supplement applications (**Figure 7**).

Globalization, innovation, and free trade have contributed to the rise of nontraditional food products across the globe. Algae-related products are one example of nontraditional food with a short history of consumption in Europe. Regulation EC 2015/2283 (formerly EC 258/97) set the boundaries and procedures for selling food products that are safe for humans and that were not consumed before May 15, 1997 [64, 65]. Therefore, products that were not present in the European market before this date are considered Novel Foods and they must be approved by following an authorization procedure. Most algal products fall under the Novel Food category, and as such, their safe consumption must be ensured. The authorized products are available in the Union List of Novel Foods, which is regularly updated (CIR EU 2017/2470) [66]. Foods that are not "Novel" are listed in the EU Novel Food status Catalog, which is a nonbinding list used for guidance purposes [67]. The presence of spirulina in the Catalog indicates that several species of spirulina were consumed in Europe before May 15, 1997.

Starting from the design phase, adequate permissions are required for the building and construction of the facilities while bearing in mind the final application of the product. Once the facility is operational, these permits must be maintained over time. The operation of the facilities requires the use of several inputs ranging from the raw materials to cultivate spirulina such as nutrients, carbon dioxide, or water to energy for culture circulation and mixing. Both the raw materials used for cultivation as well as the material of the equipment used during the process must be food grade. Finally, generated waste must be managed during the operation of the facility. Environmental regulations exist that cover all impacts of spirulina production including water [68], waste [69], and emission management. Water is the most relevant topic, and the framework is similar to aquaculture and agriculture practices. In general, EU environmental law sets principles and requirements through Directives instead of Regulations, to leave some flexibility to the member states to adopt their legislation (subsidiarity principle). On the contrary, this approach leaves stakeholders facing uneven competition and hurdles due to a lack of harmonization in the legal framework. Specially for these matters, it is therefore necessary for stakeholders to consider local regulations since it is up to the specific local competent authority to comply with EU law.

All products fit for human consumption must be safe for the consumers. The safety of spirulina is mainly determined by its purity and the absence of contaminants such as pesticides, heavy metals (EC 915/2023 [70]), or microorganisms (EC 2073/2005 [71]). The safety of the product can be ensured when the cultivation and further processing of spirulina are performed in facilities and with equipment that comply with the level of hygiene stated in EC 2002/178, and by suitably trained operators. One approach to minimize risks and ensure the quality of food product is through the application of a Hazard Analysis and Critical Control Point (HACCP) plan (EC 2004/852) [72]. Shortly, the implementation and maintenance of a HACCP plan helps in the identification of hazards, establishment of monitoring procedures and correcting measures, and documentation for tracking proper hygiene practices. Besides the HACCP system, there are other similar approaches to ensure food safety and quality such as the Good Manufacturing Practice (GMP) system. The GMP system was originally designed for safety in the pharmaceutical sector, but it is also functional in the food sector. The Codex Alimentarius CAC/RCP 1-1969 [73] is a document developed by FAO and WHO that summarizes the principles of Good Hygienic Practices (GHP) and HACCP. Also, private certifications exist such as the Good Agriculture Practices (GAP) developed by Globalg.a.p. For food applications, the HACCP system is highly advisable in Europe to grow and sell spirulina that complies with food law regulations. Nevertheless, this system is not mandatory when spirulina is only cultivated (primary sector activity), but it is mandatory when the process includes transformation such as drying and/or packaging (secondary sector, i.e., industry). The business operators play a central role in the implementation of this system since they must follow the established hygienic measures and train operators to comply with them. In addition, business employers must comply with labor safety regulations defined in directive 89/391/EEC [74].

The quality of the product is a parameter of utmost relevance for the customer, and it is not an exception for microalgae. The quality of the spirulina products is specified in technical data sheets (TDS), Certificates of Analysis (CoA), or safety data sheets. These documents include information regarding the nutritional value, the storage conditions, and other properties of the product such as the purity. The nutritional information for consumers is described in the regulation 2009/1169 [75], which clearly states all the information and labeling rules of food products. It is also a common practice to include nutritional and health claims for food products in commercial communications. Regulation 2006/1924/EC addresses the potential health and nutritional claims that can be done based on the nutritional properties of the food product [76]. The purpose of this regulation is to ensure that claims are truthful, clear, and based on scientific evidence. At the moment, there are still no approved health claims for spirulina, despite several applications being under revision.

Different certificates of quality exist that can increase the value of the product. Certification is a proof of compliance, given by a third party ("Certification body"), between the supplier and the customer, usually released on a voluntary basis in front of Standards (reference documents). Despite being voluntary, it is yet required by the customer since it has a market impact. On the opposite, regulatory compliance is mandatory, verified by Official Authorities, and has a legal impact. Different types of certifications prove that a product has been developed according to certain quality, social, environmental, or religious standards. Certification of quality in products may also aim to protect the practices, origin, and tradition of certain products in Europe and includes different types of certificates such as Organic, Protected Denomination of Origin (PDO), Protected Geographical Indication PGI, or Traditional Specialties Guarantee TSG, as stated in regulation 2012/1151 [77]. Religious Certifications such as Kosher and Halal certify that the product was produced according to Kosher and Islamic law requirements, respectively. Environmental certificates such as ASC-MSC Seaweed Standard or Demeter Biodynamic Certification [78] identify those products whose production minimizes their impact on the environment.

Among the different types of certificates, the European Organic certification is the most adopted by spirulina producers. The Organic certification guarantees that a certain product has been produced according to sustainability principles and methods that minimize the impact to the environment, protect the biodiversity, and contribute to the local farming. In that case, a European regulation states the principles and rules (EC No 2018/848) and a certification body, which can vary between European countries, evaluate the compliance of a product to organic production methods [79].

8. Conclusions and prospects

In this chapter, we have examined some aspects of spirulina cultivation. Spirulina is probably the easiest microalga to cultivate in a safe and efficient way. Compared to other microalgae, there is ample experience in cultivation and human consumption of spirulina, but the exposition in this chapter shows that we are far from agreeing even on basic terms like safety, quality, and optimal cultivation technology, even less on engineering of spirulina cultivation, harvesting, and drying systems. Part of this disagreement is rooted in biology and enormous intraspecies diversity as well as high variability of climatic and environmental conditions. Even larger part of disagreement belongs to different objective values: what is safe spirulina, does market demand organically certified cyanobacteria, what are the quality criteria of a good product, and what are legal and regulatory constraints? In short, what is the market demand?

Europe is lagging on algal production compared to other parts of the world. Spirulina has gained some market share in European markets, although the popularity of spirulina in different markets varies significantly; there are countries with decades of tradition of spirulina consumption and countries where spirulina is virtually unknown. Most of spirulina consumed in Europe is imported from various sources; some are decently good, some less so; there is almost no criteria to evaluate product quality or product value.

Spirulina cultivation is Europe cannot compete with the cost of production elsewhere—cultivation conditions, labor, and investment cost, and also, regulatory constraints in other parts of the world are simply more favorable. However, spirulina made in Europe may and must be competitive in quality, taste, local origin, branding, product safety, and environmental impact.

Variations in product quality have already raised concerns of various consumer organizations on spirulina safety [80–82]. Up to now, most of the warnings were formulated as advice to consumers to rely on reputable sources of spirulina, but the community can easily lose credibility in the eyes of the consumers. So, adhering to strict safety and quality standards to avoid heavy metal, bacterial, or cyanotoxin contamination (in the pond or after filtering) and avoidance of higher temperatures are important for the whole community. We cannot be happy to produce safe spirulina while unsafe spirulina is being on the market—consumers are prone to generalize, and they do not distinguish different production methods.

Another important conclusion of the presentations in this chapter can be summarized with a statement "scaling-up is not easy." Methods and techniques that work in the lab or even in a small pond are not directly applicable at large scale. Cleanliness and contamination prevention in the lab is usually a normal routine, while it is impossible to protect a large pond from all contaminants, even more, a contamination source is not easily discovered at large scale. This means that upscaling is a task of professionals with experience and methodology that will result in a manageable system and manageable processes.

To achieve consistent high quality and high productivity, process optimization should focus on both upstream and downstream operations. The design, safety, and quality aspects of large-scale spirulina cultivation are critical for ensuring a successful operation. The design focuses on creating a controlled environment that maximizes spirulina growth while minimizing contamination risks. Safety measures include maintaining high cleanliness standards, employing clean room technologies, and implementing safe procedures. Quality is achieved through a combination of design decisions to prevent contamination, ensure consistent nutrient distribution, and maintain nutrient integrity. These components work together to produce spirulina that is safe, of high quality, and produced efficiently on a large scale. Last but not least, best quality standards and demanding regulatory framework such as those in EU have huge impact on quality and safety of EU farmed spirulina.

The regulatory framework around a specific spirulina product is thus an aspect that must be considered at early stages. Despite lack of specific spirulina production regulation or standards, it is worth noting the use of the regulatory framework of the aquaculture sector as a reference point for stakeholders. We should consider good regulation as an asset rather than an obstacle. Clarification and awareness of the regulatory framework is important for hygiene and safety of the products, the people in the process, as well as the sustainability of the whole process.

There is more to be done at the R&D level. The recycling of water and excess nutrients plays an important role in quality, sustainability, and profitability. Based on the varying experience of different producers, more R&D work is required. Another almost untouched area is the taste of spirulina: different products come with different tastes, which is of a primary importance for consumers with no explanation what is determining the taste of the product.

A very important basis for process control is good modeling that includes relevant physical, chemical, and biological factors into a powerful process models that can be used as digital twins and predictive component of the process control algorithms. Kinetic models cannot be replaced by artificial intelligence; they may be augmented by AI in some aspects like parameter adjustments. Availability of affordable metagenomic tools seems to call for inclusion of metagenomic data into the models as a verification and parameter adjustment mechanisms. Higher level of control in very large production systems demand early warning functionality that will enable proactive controls.

Spirulina farming is frequently considered as the entry level technology to a more demanding farming of other species. Provided that spirulina market exists, it is also the safest investment prior to moving into some other higher value products. Spirulina itself is a safe and sustainable source of protein, antioxidants, and other substances that will become more and more important as replacement of other protein sources with high environmental impacts. In this view, we can consider it a strategic technology, and there is no doubt Europe has to be active in its development to reduce the lag from countries where these technologies are already developed at very large scale. We have to do it considering our own climatic, environmental, and market conditions, and it seems we can do it in a commercially viable way.

Acknowledgements

This work has been supported by the grants from Slovenian national projects EIP Mordozelena, grant L4-4564 and AlGreen J2-4427, and Horizon Europe projects BioRural (grant 101060166), Cronus (grant 101084405), FuelPhoria (grant 101118286), and Locality (grant 101112884).

DOI: http://dx.doi.org/10.5772/intechopen.1005474

Author details

Maja Berden Zrimec[1*], Eleonora Sforza[2], Leonardo Pattaro[2], Davide Carecci[3], Elena Ficara[4], Antonio Idà[5], Narcís Ferrer-Ledo[6], Stefano Canziani[6], Silvio Mangini[7], Borut Lazar[1], Sophia Papadaki[8], Giorgos Markou[9], Ioannis Tzovenis[10] and Robert Reinhardt[1]

1 Algen, Algal Technology Centre, LLC, Ljubljana, Slovenia

2 Department of Industrial Engineering, University of Padova, Italy

3 Department of Electronics, Information and Bioengineering, Politecnico di Milano, Milano, Italy

4 Department of Civil and Environmental Engineering, Politecnico di Milano, Milano, Italy

5 Algaria SRL, Milano, Italy

6 Algreen B.V., Wageningen, The Netherlands

7 Archimede Ricerche SRL, Genova, Italy

8 Department of Chemical Engineering, National Technical University of Athens, Athens, Greece

9 Institute of Technology of Agricultural Products, Hellenic Agricultural Organization, Dimitra, Lycovrysi, Greece

10 Microphykos, Athens, Greece

*Address all correspondence to: maja@algen.si

References

[1] Araújo R, Vazquez Calderon F, Sánchez Lopez J, Azevedo IC, Bruhn A, Fluch S, et al. Current status of the algae production industry in Europe: An emerging sector of the blue bioeconomy. Frontiers in Marine Science. 2021;**7**:1-24. DOI: 10.3389/fmars.2020.626389

[2] FAO. Global Seaweeds and Microalgae Production, 1950–2019. FAO Global Fishery and Aquaculture Production Statistics (FishStatJ). Rome, Italy: Food and Agriculture Organization of the United States; 2021. Available from: www.fao.org/fishery/statistics/software/fishstatj/en

[3] IMARC. Spirulina Market Report by Species (*Arthrospira Platensis, Arthrospira Maxima*) 2024–2032. New York, USA: International Market Analysis Research and Consulting Group; 2023

[4] Nowicka-Krawczyk P, Mühlsteinová R, Hauer T. Detailed characterization of the Arthrospira type species separating commercially grown taxa into the new genus *Limnospira* (cyanobacteria). Scientific Reports. 2019;**9**(1):1-11

[5] Roussel T, Halary S, Duval C, Piquet B, Cadoret JP, Vernès L, et al. Monospecific renaming within the cyanobacterial genus *Limnospira (spirulina)* and consequences for food authorization. Journal of Applied Microbiology. 2023;**134**(8): lxad159. DOI: 10.1093/jambio/lxad159

[6] Ramlee A, Rasdi NW, Abd Wahid ME, Jusoh M. Microalgae and the factors involved in successful propagation for mass production. Journal of Sustainable Science and Management. 2021;**16**:21-42. DOI: 10.46754/jssm.2021.04.003

[7] Fagiri YMA, Salleh A, El-Nagerabi SAF. Impact of physico-chemical parameters on the physiological growth of *Arthrospira* (*Spirulina platensis*) exogenous strain UTEXLB2340. AJB. 2013;**12**(35):5458-5465. DOI: 10.5897/AJB2013.12234. ISSN 1684-5315

[8] USDA (U.S. Department of Agriculture). Agricultural research service. 2024. Available from: https://fdc.nal.usda.gov/fdc-app.html#/food-details/170091/nutrients

[9] Wu L, Orikasa T, Ogawa Y, Tagawa A. Vacuum drying characteristics of eggplants. Journal of Food Engineering. 2007;**83**(3):422-429

[10] Chen CL, Huang CC, Ho KC, Hsiao PX, Wu MS, Chang JS. Biodiesel production from wet microalgae feedstock using sequential wet extraction/transesterification and direct transesterification processes. Bioresource Technology. 2015;**194**: 179-186

[11] Show KY, Lee DJ, Mujumdar AS. Advances and challenges on algae harvesting and drying. Drying Technology. 2015;**33**(4):386-394

[12] Oliveira EG, Duarte JH, Moraes K, Crexi VT, Pinto LAA. Optimisation of *Spirulina platensis* convective drying: Evaluation of phycocyanin loss and lipid oxidation. International Journal of Food Science and Technology. 2010a;**45**: 1572-1578

[13] Marques LG, Freire JT. Analysis of freeze-drying of tropical fruits. Drying Technology. 2005;**23**(9–11):2169-2184

[14] Oliveira EG, Rosa GS, Moraes MA, Pinto LAA. Phycocyanin content of *Spirulina platensis* dried in spouted bed

and thin layer. Journal of Food Process Engineering. 2008;**31**(1):34-50

[15] Kyriakopoulou K, Pappa A, Krokida M, Detsi A, Kefalas P. Effects of drying and extraction methods on the quality and antioxidant activity of sea buckthorn (*Hippophae rhamnoides*) berries and leaves. Drying Technology. 2013;**31**(9):1063-1076

[16] Šumić Z, Vakula A, Tepić A, Čakarević J, Vitas J, Pavlić B. Modeling and optimization of red currants vacuum drying process by response surface methodology (RSM). Food Chemistry. 2016;**203**:465-475

[17] Agustini TW, Suzery M, Sutrisnanto D, Ma'ruf WF. Comparative study of bioactive substances extracted from fresh and dried *Spirulina* sp. Procedia Environmental Sciences. 2015;**23**:282-289

[18] Papadaki S, Kyriakopoulou K, Stramarkou M, Tzovenis I, Krokida M. Environmental assessment of industrially applied drying technologies for the treatment of *Spirulina platensis*. IOSR Journal of Environmental Science, Toxicology and Food Technology (IOSR-JESTFT). 2017;**11**(1):41-46

[19] Stramarkou M, Papadaki S, Kyriakopoulou K, Tzovenis I, Chronis M, Krokida M. Comparative analysis of different drying techniques based on the qualitative characteristics of *Spirulina platensis* biomass. Journal of Aquatic Food Product Technology. 2021;**30**(5): 498-516. DOI: 10.1080/10498850.2021.1900969

[20] Novoveská L, Nielsen SL, Eroldoğan OT, Haznedaroglu BZ, Rinkevich B, Fazi S, et al. Overview and challenges of large-scale cultivation of photosynthetic microalgae and cyanobacteria. Marine Drugs. 2023;**21**: 445. DOI: 10.3390/MD21080445

[21] Schulze PSC, Guerra R, Pereira H, Schüler LM, Varela JCS. Flashing LEDs for microalgal production. Trends in Biotechnology. 2017;**35**:1088-1101

[22] Bertucco A, Beraldi M, Sforza E. Continuous microalgal cultivation in a laboratory-scale photobioreactor under seasonal day-night irradiation: Experiments and simulation. Bioprocess and Biosystems Engineering. 2014;**37**: 1535-1542

[23] Fernandes BD, Mota A, Teixeira JA, Vicente AA. Continuous cultivation of photosynthetic microorganisms: Approaches, applications and future trends. Biotechnology Advances. 2015; **33**:1228-1245. DOI: 10.1016/J.BIOTECHADV.2015.03.004

[24] Pastore M, Primavera A, Milocco A, Barbera E, Sforza E. Tuning the solid retention time to boost microalgal productivity and carbon exploitation in an industrial pilot-scale LED photobioreactor. Industrial and Engineering Chemistry Research. 2022; **61**:7739-7747. DOI: 10.1021/ACS.IECR.2C01031

[25] Barbera E, Sforza E, Grandi A, Bertucco A. Uncoupling solid and hydraulic retention time in photobioreactors for microalgae mass production: A model-based analysis. Chemical Engineering Science. 2020;**218**: 115578. DOI: 10.1016/J.CES.2020.115578

[26] Bernard O, Rémond B. Validation of a simple model accounting for light and temperature effect on microalgal growth. Bioresource Technology. 2012; **123**:520-527. DOI: 10.1016/J.BIORTECH.2012.07.022

[27] Peeters JCH, Eilers P. The relationship between light intensity and

photosynthesis-A simple mathematical model. Hydrobiological Bulletin. 1978;**12**: 134-136. DOI: 10.1007/BF02260714/ METRICS

[28] Platt T, Gallegos C, Harrison W. Photoinhibition of photosynthesis in natural assemblages of marine phytoplankton. Journal of Marine Research. 1980;**38**:687-701

[29] Droop MR. 25 years of algal growth kinetics: A personal view. Botanica Marina. 1983;**26**:99-112. DOI: 10.1515/ BOTM.1983.26.3.99

[30] Sforza E, Urbani S, Bertucco A. Evaluation of maintenance energy requirements in the cultivation of *Scenedesmus obliquus*: Effect of light intensity and regime. Journal of Applied Phycology. 2015;**27**:1453-1462. DOI: 10.1007/S10811-014-0460-X/ FIGURES/6

[31] Depraetere O, Pierre G, Noppe W, Vandamme D, Foubert I, Michaud P, et al. Influence of culture medium recycling on the performance of *Arthrospira platensis* cultures. Algal Research. 2015;**10**:48-54. DOI: 10.1016/J. ALGAL.2015.04.014

[32] Kurpan D, Idà A, Körner FG, Bombelli P, da Silva Aguiar JP, Marinho LM, et al. Long-term evaluation of productivity and harvesting efficiency of an industrial spirulina (*Arthrospira platensis*) production facility. Bioresource Technology Reports. 2024; **25**:101741. DOI: 10.1016/J. BITEB.2023.101741

[33] Béchet Q, Shilton A, Park JB, Craggs RJ, Guieysse B. Universal temperature model for shallow algal ponds provides improved accuracy. Environmental Science & Technology. 2011;**45**(8):3702-3709. DOI: 10.1021/ es1040706

[34] Li S, Willits DH, Browdy CL, Timmons MB, Losordo TM. Thermal modeling of greenhouse aquaculture raceway systems. Aquacultural Engineering. 2009;**41**(1):1-13. DOI: 10.1016/j.aquaeng.2009.04.002

[35] Carecci D. Thermal and biological modeling of microalgae cultivation on digestate under greenhouse in synergy with a biomethane plant [Master thesis] Politecnico di Milano. 2022. Available from: https://hdl.handle.net/10589/ 191674

[36] Rosso L, Lobry JR, Flandrois JP. An unexpected correlation between cardinal temperatures of microbial growth highlighted by a new model. Journal of Theoretical Biology. 1993;**162**(4): 447-463. DOI: 10.1006/jtbi.1993.1099

[37] Rossi S, Carecci D, Ficara E. Thermal response analysis and compilation of cardinal temperatures for 424 strains of microalgae, cyanobacteria, diatoms and other species. Science of the Total Environment. 2023;**873**:162275. DOI: 10.1016/j.scitotenv.2023.162275

[38] Casagli F, Zuccaro G, Bernard O, Steyer JP, Ficara E. ALBA: A comprehensive growth model to optimize algae-bacteria wastewater treatment in raceway ponds. Water Research. 2021;**190**:116734. DOI: 10.1016/j.watres.2020.116734

[39] Chaiklahan R, Chirasuwan N, Srinorasing T, Attasat S, Nopharatana A, Bunnag B. Enhanced biomass and phycocyanin production of *Arthrospira (Spirulina) platensis* by a cultivation management strategy: Light intensity and cell concentration. Bioresource Technology. 2022;**343**:126077. DOI: 10.1016/j.biortech.2021.126077

[40] Vonshak A, Guy R. Photoadaptation, photoinhibition and

productivity in the blue-green alga, *Spirulina platensis* grown outdoors. Plant, Cell and Environment. 1992;**15**: 613-616

[41] Kilimtzidi E, Cuellar Bermudez S, Markou G, Goiris K, Vandamme D, Muylaert K. Enhanced phycocyanin and protein content of *Arthrospira* by applying neutral density and red light shading filters: A small-scale pilot experiment. Journal of Chemical Technology and Biotechnology. 2019;**94**: 2047-2054

[42] Muys M, González Cámara SJ, Arnau C, García D, Peiro E, Gòdia F, et al. Light regime, harvesting time and operation mode can optimize the productivity of nutritional protein in *Chlorella and Spirulina* biomass. Algal Research. 2024;**79**:103443

[43] Yang Z, Xu B, Liu J, Zhan J, Song L. Dynamic changes of growth and physiological parameters of *Spirulina* cultivated outdoors—A case study in *Spirulina* Industrial Park in Inner Mongolia, China. Journal of Applied Phycology. 2022;**34**:1163-1175

[44] Markou G, Kougia E, Arapoglou D, Chentir I, Andreou V, Tzovenis I. Production of *Arthrospira platensis*: Effects on growth and biochemical composition of long-term acclimatization at different salinities. Bioengineering. 2023;**10**:233

[45] Bhakar R, Kumar R, Pabbi S. Total lipids and fatty acid profile of different spirulina strains as affected by salinity and incubation time. Vegetos. 2013;**26**: 148-154

[46] de Morais EG, Nunes IL, Druzian JI, de Morais MG, da Rosa APC, Costa JAV. Increase in biomass productivity and protein content of *Spirulina* sp. LEB 18 (*Arthrospira*) cultivated with crude glycerol. Biomass Conversion and Biorefinery. 2020;**12**(21):1-9

[47] Markou G, Kougia E, Kefalogianni I, Tsagou V, Arapoglou D, Chatzipavlidis I. Effect of glycerol concentration and light intensity on growth and biochemical composition of *Arthrospira (Spirulina) platensis*: A study in semi-continuous mode with non-aseptic conditions. Applied Sciences. 2019;**9**:4703

[48] Kougia E, Ioannou E, Roussis V, Tzovenis I, Chentir I, Markou G. Iron (Fe) biofortification of *Arthrospira platensis*: Effects on growth, biochemical composition and in vitro iron bioaccessibility. Algal Research. 2023;**70**: 103016

[49] Saeid A, Chojnacka K, Korczyński M, Korniewicz D, Dobrzański Z. Biomass of *Spirulina maxima* enriched by biosorption process as a new feed supplement for swine. Journal of Applied Phycology. 2013;**25**: 667-675

[50] Zinicovscaia I, Cepoi L, Rudi L, Chiriac T, Grozdov D, Vergel K. Effect of zinc-containing systems on *Spirulina platensis* bioaccumulation capacity and biochemical composition. Environmental Science and Pollution Research. 2021;**28**:52216-52224

[51] Markou G, Eliopoulos C, Argyri A, Arapoglou D. Production of *Arthrospira (Spirulina) platensis* enriched in β-Glucans through phosphorus limitation. Applied Sciences. 2021;**11**:8121

[52] Vonshak A, Richmond A. Mass production of the blue-green alga *Spirulina*: An overview. Biomass. 1988; **15**:233-247. DOI: 10.1016/0144-4565(88)90059-5

[53] EN 17399:2020. Algae and algae products – Terms and definitions. 2021

[54] Smith AG, Tredici MR, Boussiba S, Verdelho V, Cadoret JP, Davey MP, et al. What are Algae? [Internet]. 2021 [cited 2024 Mar 10]. Available from: https://www.what-are-algae.com/

[55] Council. Regulation (EC) No 708/2007 concerning the use of alien and locally absent species in aquaculture. Official Journal of the European Union [internet]. 11 Jun 2007;**L168**:1-17 [cited 2024 Feb 12]. Available from: https://eur-lex.europa.eu/

[56] European Parliament and the Council. Regulation (EU) No 1379/2013 on the common organisation of the markets in fishery and aquaculture products, amending Council Regulations (EC) No 1184/2006 and (EC) No 1224/2009 and repealing Council Regulation (EC) No 104/2000. Official Journal of the European Union [internet]. 11 Dec 2013; **L354**:1-21 [cited 2024 Feb 2]. Available from: https://eur-lex.europa.eu/

[57] European Parliament and the Council. Regulation (EC) No 178/2002 laying down the general principles and requirements of food law, establishing the European Food Safety Authority and laying down procedures in matters of food safety. Official Journal of the European Union. 28 Jan 2002;**L31**:1-24 [cited 2024 Feb 13]. Available from: https://eur-lex.europa.eu/

[58] European Parliament and the Council. Directive 2002/46/EC on the approximation of the laws of the Member States relating to food supplements. Official Journal of the European Communities [Internet]. 10 Jun 2002;**L183**:51-57 [cited 2024 Feb 01]. Available from: https://eur-lex.europa.eu/

[59] European Parliament and the Council. Regulation (EC) No 767/2009 of the European Parliament and of the Council of 13 July 2009 on the placing on the market and use of feed, amending European Parliament and Council Regulation (EC) No 1831/2003 and repealing Council Directive 79/373/EEC, Commission Directive 80/511/EEC, Council Directives 82/471/EEC, 83/228/EEC, 93/74/EEC, 93/113/EC and 96/25/EC and Commission Decision 2004/217/EC. Official Journal of the European Union [Internet]. 13 Jul 2009;**L229**:1-28 [cited 2024 Feb 13]. Available from: https://eur-lex.europa.eu/

[60] European Parliament and the Council. Regulation (EC) No 1223/2009 on cosmetic products. Official Journal of the European Union [Internet]. 30 Nov 2009;**L342**:59-209 [cited 2024 Feb 25]. Available from: https://eur-lex.europa.eu/

[61] European Parliament and the Council. Regulation (EU) No 2019/1009 laying down rules on the making available on the market of EU fertilising products and amending Regulations (EC) No 1069/2009 and (EC) No 1107/2009 and repealing Regulation (EC) No 2003/2003. Official Journal of the European Union [Internet]. 5 Jun 2019; **L170**:1-114 [cited 2024 Feb 22]. Available from: https://eur-lex.europa.eu/

[62] European Parliament and the Council. Directive 2001/83/EC on the Community code relating to medicinal products for human use. Official Journal of the European Communities [Internet]. 6 Nov 2001;**L311**:67-128 [cited 2024 Feb 21]. Available from: https://eur-lex.europa.eu/

[63] European Parliament and the Council. Regulation (EU) No 609/2013 of 12 June 2013 on food intended for infants and young children for special medical purposes, and total diet

replacement for weight control and repealing Council Directive 92/52/EEC, Commission Directives 96/8/EC, 1999/21/EC, 2006/125/EC, 2006/141/EC, Directive 2009/39/EC of the European Parliament and of the Council and Commission Regulations (EC) No 41/2009 and (EC) No 953/2009. Official Journal of the European Union [Internet]. 12 Jun 2013;**L181**:35-56 [cited 2024 Feb 9]. Available from: https://eur-lex.europa.eu/

[64] European Parliament and the Council. Regulation (EU) 2015/2283 on novel foods, amending Regulation (EU) No 1169/2011 of the European Parliament and of the Council and repealing Regulation (EC) No 258/97 of the European Parliament and of the Council and Commission Regulation (EC) No 1852/2001. Official Journal of the European Union [Internet]. 25 Nov 2015; **L327**:1-22 [cited 2024 Feb 16]. Available from: https://eur-lex.europa.eu/

[65] European Parliament and the Council. Regulation (EC) No 258/97 concerning novel foods and novel food ingredients. Official Journal of the European Communities [Internet]. 27 Jan 1997;**L43**:1-6 [cited 2024 Feb 10]. Available from: https://eur-lex.europa.eu/

[66] European Commission. Commission Implementing Regulation (EU) 2017/2470 establishing the Union list of novel foods in accordance with Regulation (EU) 2015/2283 of the European Parliament and of the Council on novel foods. Official Journal of the European Union [Internet]. 20 Dec 2017;**L351**:72-201 [cited 2024 Feb 4]. Available from: https://eur-lex.europa.eu/

[67] Novel Food status Catalogue. Available from: Novel Food status Catalogue - European Commission (europa.eu) [Accessed: March 22, 2024]

[68] European Parliament and the Council. Directive 2000/60/EC establishing a framework for Community action in the field of water policy. Official Journal of the European Communities. 23 Oct 2000;**L327**:1-72 [cited 2024 Feb 20]. Available from: https://eur-lex.europa.eu/

[69] European Parliament and the Council. Directive 2008/98/EC on waste and repealing certain Directives. Official Journal of the European Union [Internet]. 19 Nov 2008;**L312**:3-30 [cited 2024 Feb 23]. Available from: https://eur-lex.europa.eu/

[70] European Commission. Commission Regulation (EU) 2023/915 on maximum levels for certain contaminants in food and repealing Regulation (EC) No 1881/2006. Official Journal of the European Union [Internet]. 25 Apr 2023;**L119**:103-157 [cited 2024 Feb 23]. Available from: https://eur-lex.europa.eu/

[71] European Commission. Commission Regulation (EC) No 2073/2005 on microbiological criteria for foodstuff. Official Journal of the European Union [Internet]. 15 Nov 2005;**L338**:1-32 [cited 2024 Feb 22]. Available from: https://eur-lex.europa.eu/

[72] European Parliament and the Council. Regulation (EC) No 852/2004 on the hygiene of foodstuffs. Official Journal of the European Communities [Internet]. 29 Apr 2004;**L139**:1-25 [cited 2024 Feb 13]. Available from: https://eur-lex.europa.eu/

[73] FAO & WHO. General principles of food hygiene. Codex Alimentarius Code of Practice, No. CXC 1–1969. Codex Alimentarius Commission. Rome. 2023

[74] Council. Council Directive 89/391/EEC on the introduction of measures to encourage improvements in the safety

and health of workers at work. Official Journal of the European Communities [Internet]. 12 Jun 1989;**L183**:1-8 [cited 2024 Feb 15]. Available from: https://eur-lex.europa.eu/

[75] European Commission. Commission Regulation (EC) No 1169/2009 amending Regulation (EC) No 353/2008 establishing implementing rules for applications for authorisation of health claims as provided for in Article 15 of Regulation (EC) No 1924/2006 of the European Parliament and of the Council. Official Journal of the European Union [Internet]. 30 Nov 2009;**L314**:34-35 [cited 2024 Feb 16]. Available from: https://eur-lex.europa.eu/

[76] European Parliament and the Council. Regulation (EC) No 1924/2006 on nutrition and health claims made on foods. Official Journal of the European Union [Internet]. 20 Dec 2006;**L404**:9-25 [cited 2024 Feb 29]. Available from: https://eur-lex.europa.eu/

[77] European Parliament and the Council. Regulation (EU) No 1151/2012 on quality schemes for agricultural products and foodstuff. Official Journal of the European Union. 21 Nov 2012; L343:1-29 [cited 2024 Feb 14]. Available from: https://eur-lex.europa.eu/

[78] Biodynamic Federation Demeter. Production, Processing and Labelling. International Standard for the use and certification of Demeter, Biodynamic and related trademarks. 2023

[79] European Parliament and the Council. Regulation (EU) 2018/848 on organic production and labelling of organic products and repealing Council Regulation (EC) No 834/2007. Official Journal of the European Union [Internet]. 30 May 2018;**L150**:1-92 [cited 2024 Feb 18]. Available from: https://eur-lex.europa.eu/

[80] Großhagauer S, Kraemer K, Somoza V. The true value of *Spirulina*. Journal of Agricultural and Food Chemistry. 2020; **68**(14):4109-4115. DOI: 10.1021/acs.jafc.9b08251

[81] Thomas C, Symoneaux R, Pantin-Sohier G, Picouet P, Maître I. Perceptions of spirulina from French consumers of organic products. 2020. hal-02615769

[82] ANSES. Opinion of the French Agency for Food, Environmental and Occupational Health & Safety on the "risks associated with the consumption of food supplements containing spirulina". Request No 2014-SA-0096. 2017

Chapter 3

The Biodiversity of Algae and Physio-Chemical Parameters of the Sewage Treatment Plant and Its Canal Length, Located in Sana'a City, Yemen

Saida A. Dowman, Ashar Khalil, Sameera Y. Al-Hakmi and Nabil Al-Shwafi

Abstract

This study of the biodiversity of algae is the first interest in Yemen as a future vision for sustainable alternative solutions using sustainable resources as a sewage treatment plant with its channel length in Sana'a city, Yemen. The study aimed to screen the family of algal genera. A total of 13 samples were selected with GPS, and 100 ml of water was filled up in a plastic container and directly read as wet preparation under light microscope, identified in accordance with algae standard methods in three replicates with determination of temperature, pH, and total dissolved salts. The results showed that microalgae were conducted higher than others' algae under the mean value of temperature 28°C and neutral pH and high total dissolved salt, indicating the economical role of algae presence and waste treating by algae in despite of there was no physical or chemical processing treatment done, and the microalgae genus was found as Chlorella vulgaries with a ratio of 100%, followed by *Chlamedomonas reinhardtii and Kirchneriella lunaries* with a ratio of 76.72%, and the less found genus of filamentous algae was *Nostoc sp., Oscillatoria phucus, Ulotrix micrasterias, Dingoflagellate ceratium*, and Desmedium with a ratio of 7.69% for each, and finally, diatoms were found along the stages. The variant of the algal family will be used soon for many applications next studies.

Keywords: microalgae, biodiversity, sewage treatment plant, physicochemical parameters, biotechnological applications

1. Introduction

The algal geographical distribution is a strong indicator of large differences in the degree of their endemism and species richness in diverse regions. Information is scarce for microalgae around the world, but for some groups, some genera of algae are more endemic than others in regions of low diversity [1, 2].

Algae are a group of photosynthetic autotrophs that exist in a variety of different environments, such as lakes, rivers, seas, and sewage. They produce atmospheric oxygen through photosynthesis, which is the process of converting water and carbon dioxide into carbohydrates using solar energy in nature [3, 4]. The numerous, diverse, and high-value bioactive compounds derived from microalgae make them an important, promising, and sustainable source of beneficial bioproducts [5–7].

Microalgae contain many bioactive compounds that can be extracted and produced from their cells, including lipids, proteins, carbohydrates, carotenoids, vitamins, biodiesel, biohydrogen, biogas, and bioplastics. These bioactive compounds can be widely used in commercial, medical, and industrial applications [2, 8–11]. There are many biotechnological applications for algae in wastewater treatment plants [10]. Microalgae have significant importance for the environment. Firstly, algae have high photosynthetic efficiencies, are important as primary producers of organic matter at the base of the food chain, and provide oxygen for other aquatic life. Secondly, algae can be produced in many harsh environments not suitable for crop production, including non-arable land, saline, and wastewater. Commonly used biomasses, such as algae, also contain components such as protein, carbohydrates, and pigments [7–10, 12].

The future vision is to search for sustainable alternative solutions with friendly environmental properties that focus on algae, which is one of the available and sustainable solutions with its multiple applied uses in the fields of environment, industry, cosmetics, food supplements, medicine, etc. [13, 14]. The fact that algae are present in all environments plays an important role in the various vital processes and treatment processes [5, 15]. Therefore, this study must search for the presence of algae in this chosen environment. Therefore, the use of these effluents for the cultivation of microalgae can be interesting for the economic sustainability of the cultivation stage of algae and for environmental sustainability through the biological treatment application of the effluents forever [1, 5, 10].

Physical and chemical measurements are quantitative data that mention the presence and levels of aquatic pollution and degradation [16]. Algal aggregates are sensitive to certain pollutants that may easily accumulate within algal cells, and their metabolism within algae is also sensitive to diverse environmental and natural disturbances [17]. Several conducted studies included the presence and uses of some genus of microalgae in the effluent of wastewater and their applications, such as Nining in 2023 [18]; Mustafayeva in 2023 [19]; Senem *et al.*, in 2020 [20]; Trevore *et al.*, in 2019 [1]; Min Su., *et al.*, in 2017 [21]; Wang *et al.*, in 2016 [22]; Mahdy *et al.*, in 2016 [23]; Ebrahimian *et al.*, in 2014 [24]; Kumar and Chopra, in 2012 [25]; Borowitzka in 2013 [26]; Wang et al., in 2010 [27]; and Aach, 1952 [28]; those microalgae were *Chlorella vulgaris* and *Dunaliella* sp. And microalgae were used as renewable source for treating wastewater in the biological treatment stage as shown in the study by Wang et al. [29].

The first use of microalgae in the world dates back 2000 years to the Chinese, who used Nostoc algae during famine to survive. Microalgae biotechnology is the window to development in finding alternative and sustainable scientific solutions, which only began to appear in the middle of the last century. It has been noted that there are many commercial advertisements that use algae applications, such as microalgae in wastewater treatment [29, 30].

More studies were applied to microalgae in such applications and found to be higher than others in the classification of algae at the FB Meeting Jr. in 1996 [31].

This study of the biodiversity of algae is the first interest in Yemen as a future vision to search for sustainable alternative solutions with friendly environmental properties. In which it aimed to screen and identify the family of microalgae at the station of the sewage treatment plant and its channel length, with screening three parameters for each sample region as the primary study for more conducting studies and applications of microalgae in the area of study for wastewater treatment and other applications as soon as possible.

2. Materials and methods

2.1 Study area

The study area aimed at the Sewage Treatment Plant and its channel length during the period from the end months of the second quarter of 2021 and the first months of the third quarter of 2021 to identify the biodiversity of algae and screen three physical and chemical parameters (temperature, pH, and total dissolved salt) of the station and its channel length. As shown in the following **Figure 1**, this study targeted the sewage treatment plant located in the northern region and its channels located along the course of the sewage channel of the sewage treatment plant north of the capital, Sana'a, with an estimated length of about 20 km to the north [33]. About 95% of the irrigation crops in the study area rely on wastewater coming out of the sewage treatment plant in Sana'a that farmers use to irrigate their farms directly [33, 34]. The wastewater corridor in the Sana'a Basin starts at the outlet of the Sana'a City Wastewater Treatment Plant on the northern edge of the Sana'a Basin (Arhab and Bani al-Harith areas), and both treated and untreated sewage flows together in the channel, which is about 2.5 meters wide [35].

2.2 Sampling area

Along with the sewage treatment plant's tanks, samples were chosen to encompass nearly the whole wastewater channel stream in the research region. As shown in the accompanying **Table 1**, the sampling locations were between latitudes and longitudes of 29.5239^15'N-36.3065^15'N and 044.134912^ÍE- 04414.8938^ÍE.

2.3 Collection of water samples

Glass, polyethylene, and plastic bottles are non-sterile, hygienic, dry, and leak-proof [36]. The following procedures were used in this investigation when collecting the sample collection: Water samples should be sent as soon as possible after collection to the laboratory. Testing for algae needs to start as soon as possible after the water samples are collected, to provide the most reliable findings.

2.3.1 Analysis of the water samples microbiologically and physically

100 ml of water was filled up in a plastic container under a tightly closed and directly read as wet preparation under a light microscope with 5×, 10×, and 40× lenses times 10× according to the phycology and algae method in three replicates with determination of pH and total dissolved salts and temperature, which calculate the mean value [37, 38].

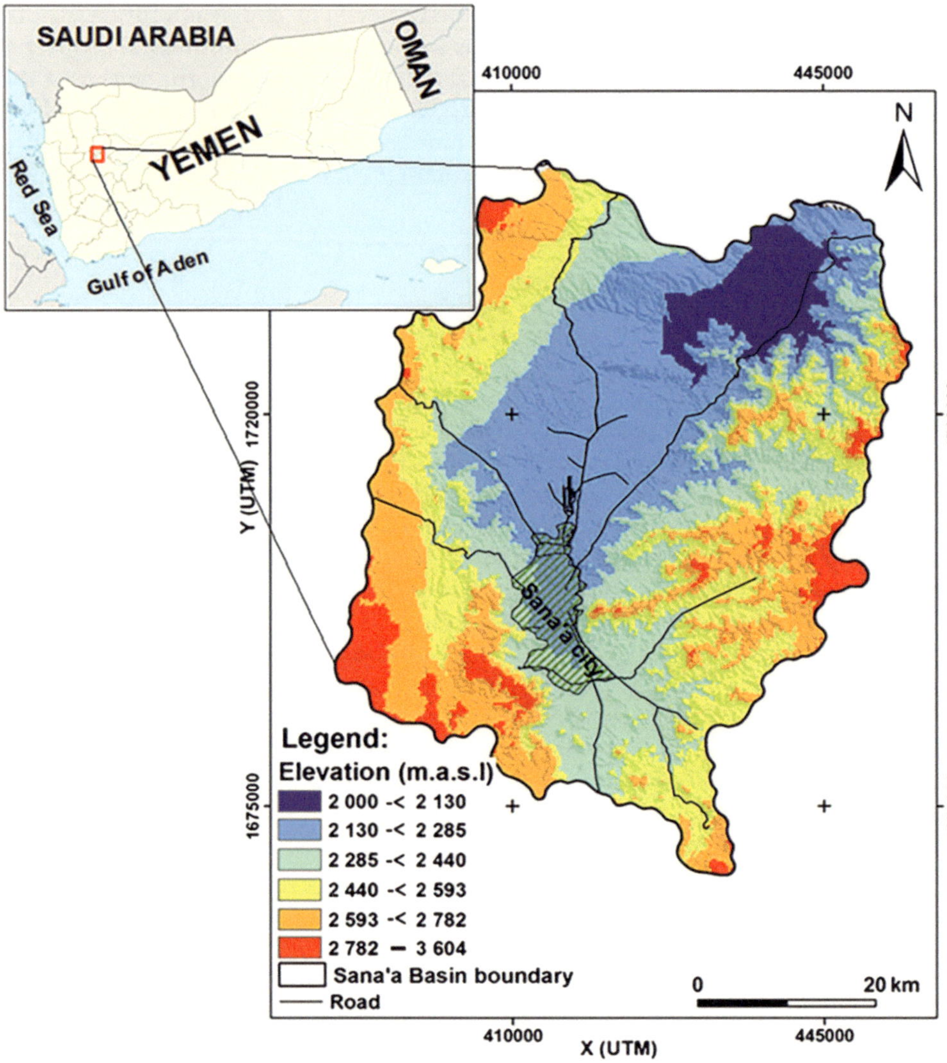

Figure 1.
Location and topographic map of the Sana'a basin Basin (study area) [digital elevation map from a satellite dataset [32].

3. Results and discussion

Table 2 shows the presence of algae that belong to the Chlorophyceae class which is seen under light microscopic examination by direct wet perpetration which shows *Chlorella vulgaris* with ratio 100% among all collected samples, followed by *Chlamedomonas reinhardtii* and *Kirchneriella lunaries* with ratio 76.92% and the less found genus of filamentous algae was *Nostoc sp., Oscillatoria phucus, Ulotrix micrasterias, Dingoflagellate ceratium, Desmedium* with ratio 7.69% for each, with the mean value of temperature 28°C; pH and total dissolved solids (TDS) were detected as shown in above table in three replicates with the mean value which shows naturalized media around 7.2 for most samples area under study and high resembles the content of TDS that appeared no treatment was done during the length of sewage channel at

Sample region		**Sample No.**	**Type of region**	**latitudes**	**longitudes**
Collection sample of aeration tanks		1	Aeration tank	29.5239°15'N	044.134912°"E
Collection sample of sedimentation tanks	WWTP-Sana'a(Sana'a wastewater treatment plant)	2	sedimentation tanks	29.8071°15'N	04413.5310°"E
drying beds		3	drying beds	29.8298°15'N	04413.5221°"E
Swamp channel initiation 1	regions along wastewater channel in Bani Alhareth and Arhab	4	wastewater pond along sewage channel Sewage	29.2856°15'N	04413.8727°"E
Swamp channel initiation 2		5		29.3086°15'N	04413.8771°"E
Swamp channel initiation 3		6		29.5045°15'N	04413.8618°"E
Bait alhellali		7		29.5910°15'N	04413.7606°"E
Bait alqaidi		8		29.6273°15'N	04413.7595°"E
Bait Quhaim		9		29.6590°15'N	04413.7450°"E
Bait handhal		10		29.8841°15'N	04413.6110°"E
Bait senhoub		11		30.0009°15'N	04413.6035°"E
Bait Haroon		12		32.8591°15'N	04413.5365°"E
Alssama Dam		13		36.3065°15'N	04414.8938°"E

Table 1.
Collected sample regions.

that year 2021 during the sample collection. The majority of the microalgae found in this study were similar to those found in the majority of the numerous studies that were conducted which play an important role in treating wastewater, as previously mentioned in reviews and literature, which discovered that Cyanobacteria—such as *Chlorella vulgaris*, *Chlamedomonas reinhardtii*, and *Cladophora sp*.—were the most common algae in sewage treatment plants across numerous stages. These algae were also used in numerous biotechnology applications, as reported by Hunter-Cevera et al. in 1996 [39], and Abdel-Raouf et al. in 2012 [40]. Moreover, comparable studies have been conducted that reported the presence of a particular genus of microalgae in wastewater effluent, wherever it was discovered. Examples of these studies include those conducted by Wang et al. in 2016 [22]; Ebrahimian et al. in 2014 [24]; Mahdy et al. in 2016 [23]; and Cabanelas et al. in 2013 [41]; Ardal in 2014 [42]; El-Sheekh et al. in 2012 [43]; Gao et al. in 2011 [44]; Min Su et al. in 2017 [21]; Senem O. C., et al., in 2020 [20] who discovered a Chlorella vulgaris, which is similar to the results of the present study. As well as a genus of *Scendesmus obliquus* mentioned in some studies done by Zhang *et al*., in 2014 and 2015 [45, 46]; Ruiz Martin *et al*., in 2010 [47]; Santos in 2017 [48]; Papazi et al. in 2013 [49]; Sethunathan et al. in 2004 [50]; and a genus of *Chlamedomonas renhardtii* mentioned in the following studies done by Su et al. in 2012 [51]; Hom-Diaz et al. in 2015 [52]; Wan et al. in 2020 [53]; Xie et al. in 2020 [54]. Although Diatoms were found in some studies done by Franziska Hempel et al. in 2011 [55] in Germany and Min Su et al. in 2017 [21]. In addition to the

Sample No.	Replicate	mean pH value	mean TDS value	Read samples in collective
1	3	7.2	876	*Chlorella vulgaris, Cosmarium spp., Cladophora surirella, Dunaliella salina, spirulina sp. Scendesmus spp. Paramecium sp., Nostoc sp. Chlamedomonas reinhardtii, Dingoflagellate ceratium, Desmedium, Gleocapsa, Oscillatoria phucus Ulotrix micrasterias.*
2	3	7.2	876	*Chlorella vulgaris, Cosmarium spp., Cladophora surirella, Dunaliella salina, Scendesmus spp. Paramecium sp., Chlamedomonas reinhardtii, Desmedium, Kirchneriella lunaries*
3	3	7.3	876	*Chlorella vulgaris, Cosmarium contructum, Chlamedomonas reinhardtii, Paramecium sp., Gleocapsa sp., Kirchneriella lunaries.*
4	3	7.2	877	*Chlorella vulgaris, Cosmarium contructum, Chlamedomonas reinhardtii, Paramecium sp., Gleocapsa sp., Kirchneriella lunaries.*
5	3	7.2	874	*Chlorella vulgaris, Cosmarium contructum, Kirchneriella lunaries.*
6	3	7.2	875	*Chlorella vulgaris, Chlamedomonas reinhardtii, Kirchneriella lunaries, Cylindrical clostridia*
7	3	7.2	876	*Chlorella vulgaris, Spirulina sp., Chlamedomonas rettenhei*
8	3	7.4	873	*Chlorella vulgaris, Spirulina sp., Chlamedomonas rettenhei*
9	3	7.2	869	*Chlorella vulgaris, Cosmarium contructum, Kirchneriella lunaries.*
10	3	7.2	868	*Chlorella vulgaris, Cosmarium contructum, Chlamedomonas reinhardtii, Paramecium sp., Gleocapsa sp., Kirchneriella lunaries.*
11	3	7.2	870	*Chlorella vulgaris, Cosmarium contructum, Kirchneriella lunaries.*
12	3	7.3	874	*Chlorella vulgaris, Chlamedomonas reinhardtii, Kirchneriella lunaries, Cylindrical clostridia*
13	3	7.2	872	*Chlorella vulgaris, Chlamedomonas reinhardtii, Kirchneriella lunaries, Cylindrical closteridia*

Table 2.
Shows the presence of microalgae and three parameters of each sample region.

same findings from the last conducted studies, others in Australia, the USA, Thailand, Taiwan, and Mexico mentioned using microalgae in biotechnology [56–61]. As well as a genus of *Scendesmus obliquus* mentioned in some studies done by Seyedeh et al. in 2021 [62]. Another similar finding was found in the following studies done by Kumar and Chopra in 2012 [25] and Palmer in 1974 [63]; Santos in 2017 [48]; Papazi et al. in 2013 [49]; Sethunathan et al. in 2004 [50] with finding a genus of *Chlamedomonas renhardtii* which was also used in many applications in the following studies done by Palmer in 1974 [64]; Mohammed in 1994 [65]; Hom-Diaz et al. in 2015 [52]; and Wan et al. in 2020 [53]. Although Diatoms isolated from wastewater were used in bioplastic applications done by Min Su et al. 2017 [21]; Franziska Hempel et al. 2011 [55] in Germany; Pittman et al. 2011 [63]; and Amos., [65], more studies should be done on the findings on microalgae not only for treating sewage water but for other applications that can be done in the future.

4. Conclusion

The findings appeared to indicate that the role of algae presence in the study area in despite of no treatment has been done on the Sana'a Sewage Treatment Plant of the area regarding the high TDS detected along the channel which need more studies to use algae presence for right treatment of wastewater, which will surely treat wastewater and decrease the causes of many diseases for human that deal with direct use of the channel either with using for irrigation of plants or farmers along the channel where there are no adding any aeration or supportive methods for irrigation of plants and farmers along the channel where there are no adding any aeration or supportive methods for getting beneficial from such algae grown as blooms on the surface of the channel as natural treatment which should be used for near future applications in area. Another point of view is that more available microalgae can be used in many applications, such as using the station for energy sources such as biofuel, biogas, biohydrogen, and so on, as well as for purifying sewage water using more microalgae.

5. Recommendation

- More attention is being paid to the economic role of microalgae in the treatment of sewage treatment plants to purify outlet sewage before exiting the channel through the sea pond in Sana'a STP.

- More studies should be done all the time to draw from natural resources and exploit them in practical applications for wastewater treatment and other uses.

- More investments in the study area for biotechnology applications are more needed.

Acknowledgements

We have to thank all the workers in the Sewage Treatment Plant who supported us for this study and did the experimental tests at their laboratory, and we have to mention that.

Conflicts of study

No financial support has been found for this study; we personally support it. There were some laboratory systems and apparatus not working, such as the BOD incubator, so we could not do other parameters.

Appendix

Some photos of selected regions of sampling and microalgae finding under microscopic lenses (5x;10x;40x) (**Figure A1**).

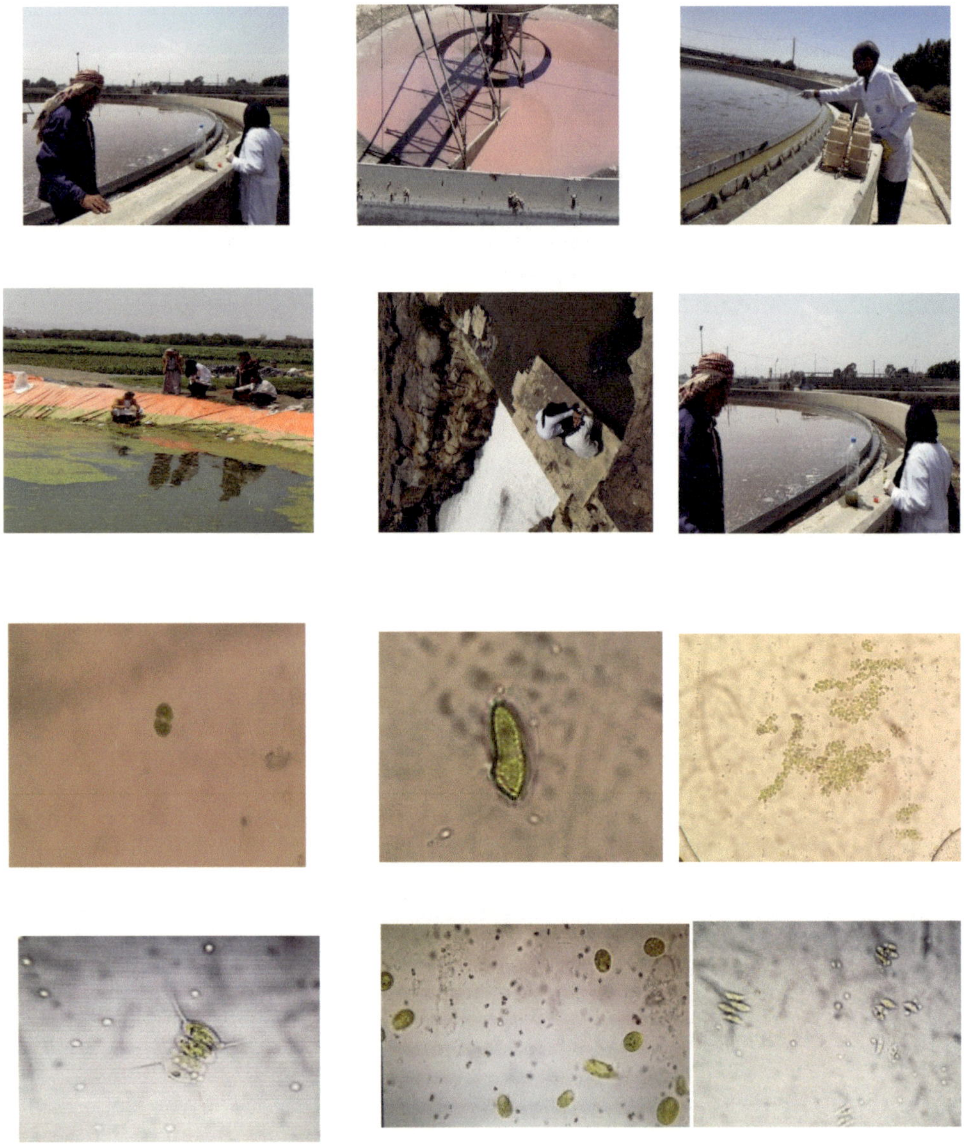

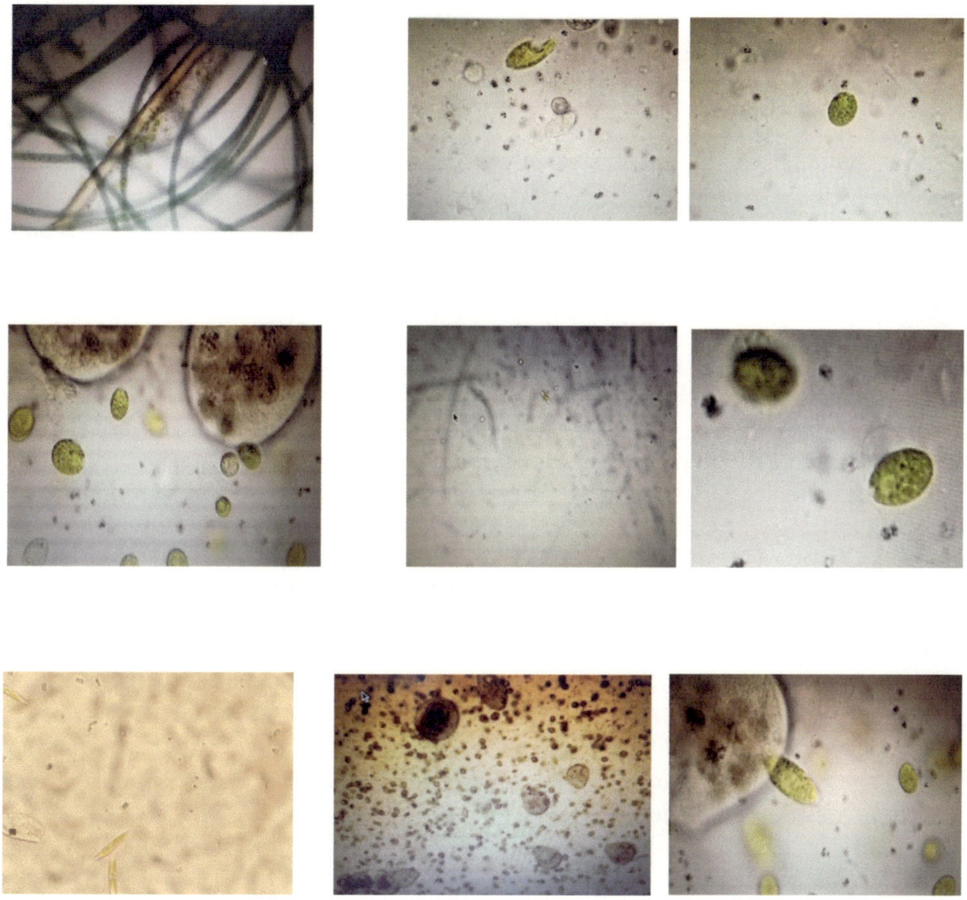

Figure A1.
Some photos of selected regions of sampling and microalgae finding under microscopic lenses (5x;10x;40x).

Author details

Saida A. Dowman[1*], Ashar Khalil[2], Sameera Y. Al-Hakmi[3] and Nabil Al-Shwafi[1]

1 Faculty of Petroleum and Natural Resources, Department of Environmental Sciences, Sana'a University, Yemen

2 Faculty of Science, Plant Section, Biology Department, Sana'a University, Yemen

3 Faculty of Science, Microbiology Section, Biology Department, Sana'a University, Yemen

*Address all correspondence to: saidadowman@ymail.com

References

[1] Norton TA, Melkonian M, Anderson RA. Algal biodiversity. Phcologia. 1994;**35**(4):308-326. DOI: 10.2216/iO031-8884-35-4-308.1

[2] Ianora A, Boersma M, Casotti R, Fontana A, Harder J, Hoffmann F, et al. New trends in marine chemical ecology. Estuaries and Coasts. 2006;**29**:531-551

[3] Singh AR, Rai PK, Sharma NK. Biodiversity and biogeography of microalgae with food and feed potential. Chapter (2). In: Hand book of Food and Feed from Microalgae, Production, Application, Regulation, and Sustainability. Academic Press; 2023. pp. 9-21. DOI: 10.1016/B978-0-323-99196-4.00038-3

[4] Guruvayoorappan C, Kuttan G. β-carotene inhibits tumor-specific angiogenesis by altering the cytokine profile and inhibits the nuclear translocation of transcription factors in B16F-10 melanoma cells. Integrative Cancer Therapies. 2007;**6**(3):258-270. DOI: 10.1177/1534735407305978

[5] Rodríguez-Roque MJ, Flores-Córdova MA, Salas-Salazar NA, Caballero MCS, ValdiviaNájar CG, Sánchez-Vega R. Microalgae as source of bioaccessible and bioavailable compound. Chapter 39. In: Hand Book of Food and Feed from Microalgae. Academic Press; 2023. pp. 519-527. DOI: 10.1016/B978-0-323-99196-4.00016-4

[6] Ikram SF, Singh L, Kumar D, et al. Prospects and constraints in studying the biodiversity of agriculturally important microalgae and cyanobacteria and useful statistical tools. Biodiversity and Conservation. 2022;**31**:1095-1124. DOI: 10.1007/s10531-022-02388-8

[7] Tanb JS, Leec SY, Chewd KW, Lame MK, Limf JW, Hoh S-H, et al. A review on microalgae cultivation and harvesting, and their biomass extractionprocessing using ionic liquids. Bioengineered. 2020;**11**(1):116-129. DOI: 10.1080/21655979.2020.1711626. Available from: http://creativecommons.org/licenses/by/4.0/

[8] Toniolo C, Nicoletti M. Quality control of microalgae-derived products. Chapter 43. In: Hand Book of Food and Feed from Microalgae, Production, Application, Regulation, and Sustainability. Available online 23 June 2023, Version of Record 23 June, Academic Press; 2023. pp. 567-575. DOI: 10.1016/B978-0-323-99196-4.00016-4

[9] Bux F, Chisti Y. Fuel alcohols from microalgae. In: Ellis JT, Miller CD, editors. Handbook of Algae Biotechnology Products and Processes. Fuel Alcohols From Microalgae. Springer; 2016. pp. 150-151

[10] The National Academies of Sciences. Sustainable Development of Algal Biofuels in the Unitated States. Washington, D.C., Available from: www.nap.edu: The National Academies of Sciences; 2012 www.national-academies.org

[11] Pilla S. Engineering applications of bioplastics and biocomposites. An overview. Handbook of Bioplastic and Biocomosites Engineering Applications. Scrivener publishing LLC. Co-published by John Wiley and Sons, in Canada. Part 1. 2011. pp. 1-15

[12] Ciferri O. Spirulina, the edible microorganism. Microbiological Reviews. 1983;**47**(4):551-578

[13] Hu I. Production of potential coproducts from microalgae. In: Biomass, Biofuels and Biochemicals. 2nd ed. Vol. 2019. Chennai, India: Elsevier; 2019. pp. 345-358. ISBN 9780444641922

[14] Jha RK, Zi-rong X. Biomedical compounds from marine organisms. Marine Drugs. 2004;**2**:123-146

[15] Stegmann P, Londo M, Junginger M. The circular bioeconomy: Its elements and role in European bioeconomy clusters. Resources, Conservation & Recycling X. 2020;**2020**(6):100029

[16] Karr JR, Chu EW. Restoring Life in Running Waters: Better Biological Monitoring. Washington DC: Island Press; 1999

[17] Stevenson RJ, Pan Y. Assessing ecological conditions in rivers and streams with diatoms. In: Stoemer EF, Smol JP, editors. The Diatom: Applications to the Environmental and Earth Science. Cambridge, UK: Cambridge University Press; 1999. pp. 11-40

[18] Nining BP. The role of indonesian indigenous cyanobacteria culture collection as an ex-situ conservation effort and Microalgae Biodiversity study material. Journal of Research in Science Education. JPPIPA; 2023;**9**(3):1269-1276. Available from: http://jppipa.unram.ac.id/index.php/jppipa/index

[19] Mustafayeva MI. Qualitative and quantitative composition of biodiversity in the ponds based on the species composition of algae. International Interdisplinary Research Journal. 2023;**2**(2):117-121. ISSN: 2835-3013. Available from: http://univerpubl.com/index.php/synergy

[20] Senem OC, Zhi KC, Mehmet AK, Nils W, Ugur C, Kerstin K. Bioplastic production from microalgae: A review. International Journal of Environmental Research and Public Health. 2020;**2020**(17):3842. DOI: 10.3390/ijerph17113842. Available from: www.mdpi.com/Journal/ijerph

[21] Min S, D'Imporzano G, Veronesiv D, Afric S, Adani F. Phaeodactylum tricornutum cultivation under mixotrophic conditions with glycerol supplied with ultrafiltered digestate: A simple biorefinery approach recovering C and N. Journal of Biotechnology. 2017;**323**(10):73-81. DOI: 10.016/J.jbiotec.2020.07.018

[22] Wang M, Yang H, Ergas SJ, vander Steen P. A novel short cut nitrogen removal process using an algal bacterial consortium in a photo-sequencing batch reactor (PSBR). Water Research. 2015;**87**:38-48

[23] Mahdy M, Aahmed A. Biological tools to improve biogas production from microalgae biomass [Thesis]. King Juan Carlos University; 2016. Available from: http://hdl.handle.net/10115/14241

[24] Ebrahimian A, Kariminia H-R, Vosoughi M. Lipid production in mixotrophic cultivation of *Chlorella vulgaris* in a mixture of primary and secondary municipal waste-water. Renewable Energy. 2014;**71**:502-508

[25] Kumar V, Chopra AK. Monitoring of physicochemical and microbiological characterstics of municipal wastewater at treatment plant, Haridwar city (Uttarakhand) India. Journal of Environmental Sciences and Technology. 2012;**5**:109-118

[26] Borowitzka MA. Energy from microalgae: A short history. Algae for biofuels and energy. Developments in Applied Phycology. Dordrecht, Netherlands: Springer; 2013;**5**:1-15.

DOI: 10.1007/978-94-007-5479-9_1. ISBN: 978-94-007-5478-2

[27] Wang L, Min M, Li Y, Chen P, Chen Y, Liu Y, et al. Cultivation of green algae chlorella sp. in different wastewaters from municipal wastewater treatment plant. Applied Biochemistry and Biotechnology. 2010;**162**:1174-1186

[28] Aach HG. Über Wachstum und Zusammensetzung von Chlorella pyrenoidosa bei unterschiedlichen Lichtstärken und Nitratmengen. Archiv für Mikrobiologie. 1952;**17**(1-4):213-246. DOI: 10.1007/BF00410827. S2CID 7813967

[29] Wang Y, Ho SH, Cheng C-L, Guo W-Q, Dilliran N, Ren NQ, et al. Perspectives on the feasibility of using microalgae for industrial wastewater treatment. Biorsourcetechnology. 2016;**222**:485-449

[30] Priyadarshani I, Rath B. Commercial and industrial applications of micro algae – A review. Journal of Algal Biomass Utilization. 2012;**3**(4):89-100. ISSN: 2229-6905

[31] Meeting FB Jr. Biodiversity and application of microalgae. Journal of Industrial Microbiology. 1996;**17**: 477-489

[32] Abdulla F, Alssa'ad T. Modelling of ground water flow for Mujib aquifer, Jordan. Journal of Earth System Science. 2006;**115**(3):289-297

[33] Merghem KA, Gharbi E, El Halouaui H, Taupin JD, Ghalit M, Alnedhary AA, et al. Quality study of wastewater treated by waste water treatment plant (WWTP) in the city of Sana'a (Yemen) used for agriculture Department of Chemistry. Faculty of Khawlan, Sana'a University, Yemen Chemistry. 2016;**4**(3):814-829

[34] Al-Sharabee R. The Effect of Using Wastewater on Microbiological Pollution for Vegetable Crops [Thesis]. Yemen: Faculty of Agriculture, Sana'a university; 2009

[35] Hydrosult I. Counsultants, Esperts-Coselis Wastewater and Sewage Sludge Reuse Feasibility Study. Yemen: Sana'a basin; 2003

[36] U.S. Environmental Protection Agency Science and Ecosystem Support Division Athens, Georgia. SESD Operating Procedure Wastewater Sampling (306)-AF. R. Athens, Georgia: U. S. Environmental Protection Agency Science and Ecosystem Support Division; 2013

[37] (APHA) Washington, D. C., American Public Health Association. Standards Methods for the Examination of Water and Wastewater. 18th ed. Washington, D.C.: (APHA), American Water Works Association (AWWA); 1998; 1975; 1985

[38] Barsanti L, Gualtieri P. Chapter 1. Algae. In: Anatomy, Biochemistry, and Biotechnology. CRC Press; 1952

[39] Hunter-Cevera JC, Jeffeies TW, Eveleigh DE. Biodiversity and application of microalgae. Journal of Industrial Microbiology and Biotechnology, ISSN: 1367-5435. 1996;**17**(5/6):477-489

[40] Abdel-Raouf N, Ibraheem IBM, Hammoida O. Eutrophication of river Nile as indicator of pollution. In: Al-Azhar Bull. Of Sci., Proceeding of 5th Int. Sci. Conf. 25-27 March 2003. 2003. pp. 293-306

[41] Cabanelas ITD, Ruiz J, Arbib Z, Chinalia FA, Garrido-Pérez C, Rogalla F, et al. Comparing the use of different domestic wastewaters for coupling microalgal production and nutrient

removal. Bioresource Technology. 2013;**131**:429-436

[42] Ardal E. Phycoremediation of Pesticides Using Microalgae [Thesis]. Sweden: Swedish University of Agricultural Sciences; 2014

[43] El-Sheekh MM, Ghareib GW, Abou-El-Souod. Biodegradation of phenolic and polycyclic aromatic compounds by some algae and cyanobacteria. Journal of Bioremediation & Biodegradation. 2012;**3**(1):133

[44] Gao QT, Wong YS, Tam NFY. Removal and biodegradation of nonylphenol by different chlorella species. Marine Pollution Bulletin. 2011;**63**(5-12):445-451

[45] Zhang T-Y, Wu Y-H, Hu H-Y. Domestic wastewater treatment and biofuel production by using microalga Scenedesmus sp. ZTY1. Water Science and Technology. 2014;**69**:2492-2496

[46] Zhang SS, Liu H, Fan JF, Yu H. Cultivation of Scenedesmus dimorphus with domestic secondary effluent and energy evaluation for biodiesel production. Environmental Technology. 2015;**36**:929-936

[47] Ruiz-Marin A, Mendoza-Espinosa LG, Stephenson T. Growth and nutrient removal in free and immobilized green algae in batch and semi-continuous cultures treating real wastewater. Bioresource Technology. 2010;**101**:58-64

[48] Santos CE, de Coimbra RN, Bermejo SP, Perez AIG, Cabero MO. Comparative assessment of pharmaceutical removal from wastewater by the microalgae Chlorella sorokiniana, Chlorella vulgaris and Scenedesmus obliquus. In: Biological Wastewater Treatment and Resource Recovery. Vol. 99. London, UK: Intechopen; 2017

[49] Papazi A, Kotzabasis K. "Rational" management of dichlorophenols biodegradation by the microalga Scenedesmus obliquus. PLoS One. 2013;**8**(4):e61682

[50] Sethunathan N, Megharaj M, Chen ZL, Williams BD, Lewis G, Naidu R. Algal degradation of a known endocrine disrupting insecticide, α-endosulfan, and its metabolite, endosulfan sulfate, in liquid medium and soil. Journal of Agricultural and Food Chemistry. 2004;**52**(10):3030-3035

[51] Su Y, Mennerich A, Urban B. Synergistic cooperation between wastewater-born algae and activated sludge for wastewater treatment: Influence of algae and sludge inoculationratios. Bioresource Technology. 2012;**105**:67-73

[52] Hom-Diaz A, Llorca M, Rodríguez-Mozaz S, Vicent T, Barcelo D, Anquez PB. Microalgae cultivation on wastewater digestate: β-estradioland17α-ethynylestradiol degradation and transformation product sidentification. Journal of Environmental Management. 2015;**155**:106-113

[53] Wan L, Wu Y, Ding H, Zhang W. Toxicity, biodegradation, and metabolic fate of organophosphorus pesticide trichlorfon on the freshwater algae, *Chlamydomonas reinhardtii*. Journal of Agricultural and Food Chemistry. 2020, 2020;**68**(6):1645-1653

[54] Xie P, Chen C, Zhang C, Su G, Ren NQ, Ho SH. Revealing the role of adsorption in ciprofloxacin and sulfadiazine elimination routes in microalgae. Water Research. 2020;**172**:115475

[55] Hempel F, Bozarth AS, Lindenkamp N, Klingl A, Zauner S, UweLinne AS, et al. Microalgae

as bioreactors for bioplastic production. Microbial Cell Factories. 2011;**10**:81. Available from: http://www.microbialcellfactories.com/content/10/1/81

[56] Borowitzka MA, Borowitzika LJ. Microalgal Biotechnology. Cambridge: Cambridge Univ. Press; 1988

[57] Borowitzka LJ, Borowitzika MA. Carotene (Provitamin a) production with algae. In: Vandamme EJ, editor. Biotechnology of Vitamins, Pigments and Growth Factors. London: Elsevier Applied Science; 1989. pp. 15-26

[58] Moreno A, Rueda O, Cabrera E, Luna-del-Castillo JD. Standaridazation in wastewater biomass growth. Facultad de Medecina, Universidad de Granada, 18012 Granada, Spain. Igiene Moderna; 1990;**94**(1):24-32

[59] Wong PK, Chan KY. Growth and value of chlorella Salina grown on highly salina sewage effluent. Agriculture, Ecosystems and Environment. 1990;**30**(3-4):334-250

[60] Renaud SM, Parry DL, Thinh LV. Microalgae for use in tropical aquaculture. 1. Gross chemical and fatty acid composition of twelve species of microalgae from the northern territory, Australia. Journal of Applied Phycology. 1994;**6**(3):337-345

[61] Borowitzka LJ, Borowitzika MA. Industrial production. Methods and economics. In: Cresswell RC, Rees TAV, Shah N, editors. Algae and Cynobacterial Biotechnology. London: Longman Scientific; 1989. pp. 244-316

[62] Seyedeh FM, Sebastian H, Nicholas W, Adebayo A, Tony G. Integrating micro-algae into wastewater treatment: A review. Science of the Total Environment. 2021;**752**:142168

[63] Pittman JK, Dean AP, Osundeko O. The potential of sustainable algal biofuel production using wastewater resources. Bioresource Technology. 2011;**102**(1):17-25. DOI: 10.1016/j.biortech.2010.06.035

[64] Palmer CM. Algae in American sewage stabilization's ponds. Revista de Microbiologia. 1974;**(S-Paulo) 5**:75-82

[65] Richmond A, Emeritus QH. Part 1. The microalgal cell. In: Hand Book of Microalgal Culture Applied Phycology and Biotechnology. 2nd ed. Vol. 3, 4. 2013. pp. 11-13

Chapter 4

Klamath Lake *Aphanizomenon Flos-Aquae*: Wild-Harvesting, Extracts and Benefits

Stefano Scoglio and Gabriel Dylan Scoglio

Abstract

This chapter examines Aphanizomenon flos-aquae (AFA) from Oregon's Klamath Lake, emphasizing its nutritional richness and health benefits. Thriving in a unique volcanic ecosystem, this wild-harvested cyanobacterium is a powerhouse of nutrients, making it a prime focus in the health supplement domain. The chapter highlights AFA's comprehensive nutritional profile, packed with proteins, essential amino acids, vitamins, minerals, and bioactive compounds. Special attention is given to AphaMax® and Klamin®, two AFA extracts with significant nutraceutical potential. AphaMax®, rich in AFA-phycocyanins, shows strong antioxidant, anti-inflammatory, wound-healing and anti-cancer properties. Klamin®, containing β-phenylethylamine (PEA), is notable for its mental health benefits, particularly in alleviating depression and anxiety, and shows promise in ADHD treatment and neurodegenerative disease management. In essence, the chapter underscores the importance of AFA from Klamath Lake as a key natural resource in the nutritional supplement industry, owing also to its potent health-promoting extracts.

Keywords: Aphanizomenon flos-aquae, Aphanizomenon, AFA, Klamath, phycocyanin, nostoc, filamentous, wild harvesting

1. Introduction

Cyanobacteria, also commonly known as blue-green algae, constitute a diverse group of ancient photoautotrophic prokaryotes [1]. These photosynthetic life forms played a pivotal role in Earth's evolutionary history during the oxygenic revolution around 2.5 billion years ago, contributing significantly to the release of oxygen into the atmosphere [2]. Displaying a remarkable diversity of morphological forms, cyanobacteria range from unicellular entities, like *Synechococcus sp.,* to intricate filaments, exemplified by *Anabaena sp.,* and colonial structures, found in *Microcystis sp.* [3]. Furthermore, these microorganisms have adapted to a wide array of habitats, from freshwater bodies, like *Planktothrix sp*., to oceans, like *Trichodesmium sp.*, to terrestrial and desert-like ones, as observed with *Chroococcidiopsis sp* [3].

Beyond their ecological significance, cyanobacteria have been studied for various applications, such as for the production of biofuel or for wastewater treatment [4, 5].

However, it is in the realm of nutritional and nutraceutical supplements that cyanobacteria truly shine. *Athrospira sp.*, colloquially known as *Spirulina*, has gained prominence as a nutritional powerhouse and has become a staple in the health supplement industry [6]. Its nutritional density and ability to be cultivated in open ponds/photobioreactors make it an attractive choice for those seeking dietary enhancements [6]. Beyond *Spirulina*, a singular *Aphanizomenon flos-aquae (AFA)* strain, Klamath *AFA*, has carved its niche in the supplement industry, owing to its superior nutritional and nutraceutical benefits, and it is directly harvested wild from Upper Klamath Lake (UKL), in Oregon, U.S.A [7].

Klamath *AFA* is a nitrogen-fixing obligate phototroph composed of cylindrical cells that self-assemble into filaments (**Figure 1**) [7]. It finds its taxonomical place within the order of the *Nostocales* and is the only *Nostocales* strain, alongside a few *Nostoc sp.*, like *N. commune* and *N. flaggeliforme*, to be regularly consumed as a dietary supplement [8, 9]. *AFA* is well known for forming fascicles, filaments that self-aggregate together into leaf-like structures which can be observed with the naked eye [7]. Furthermore, unlike *Spirulina*, *AFA* features specialized vegetative cells, known as heterocysts, which house the active nitrogenase enzyme responsible for converting atmospheric nitrogen (N^2) into ammonia [10]. Additionally, *AFA* forms akinetes, dormant cells that serve as spore-like structures, allowing the cyanobacterium to withstand unfavorable conditions and germinate into new vegetative cells when environmental conditions become favorable again [11].

AFA thrives in nutrient-rich lakes or ponds, which contribute is its ability to form blooms, dense mats of biomass that blanket the surface of lakes. Particularly renowned are the Klamath *AFA* blooms that grace UKL in Oregon, USA [7]. It is this biomass that is then harvested, processed and distributed as a nutritional supplement across the planet. UKL is the only lake in the world to be harvested for *AFA* and *AFA* is the only commercially distributed cyanobacterial supplement to be harvested from the wild at an industrial scale [12].

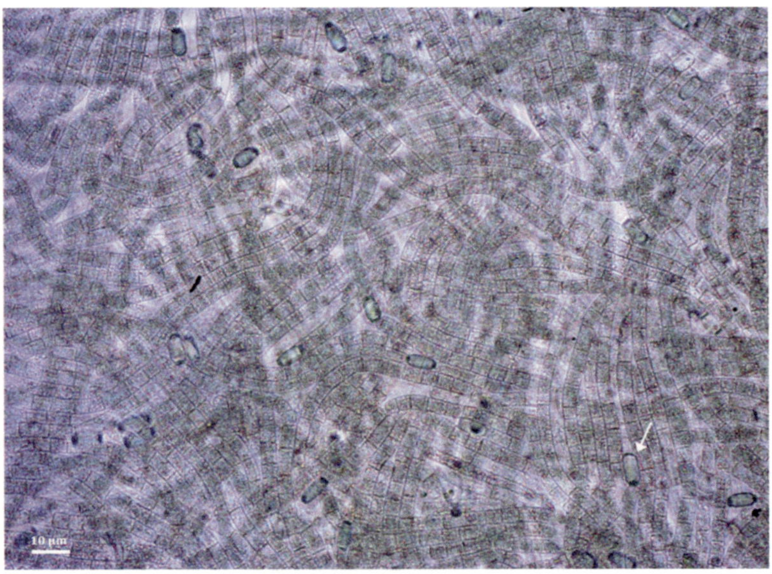

Figure 1.
Microscope image of a Klamath AFA fascicle, illustrating AFA filaments, each of which is composed by cylindrical vegetative cells. The white arrow indicates a heterocyst. Magnification: 40×.

AFA boasts a comprehensive nutritional profile: it is rich in proteins, up to 70% of total biomass, containing high amounts of all essential amino acids [9]. It contains all the vitamins, many of which at high concentration. It's a good source of polyunsaturated fatty acids (PUFAs), circa 75% of which are made of anti-inflammatory Omega-3 s [13]. Finally, thanks to the mineral richness of Klamath Lake's sediment, *AFA* provides 73 bioavailable minerals, including the complete spectrum of trace minerals [12]. The distinct biochemical profile of this substance is characterized by the presence of bioactive molecules. These include a spectrum of carotenoids, including the main xanthophylls, and an abundant concentration of chlorophyll [12]. Additionally, it contains a unique form of *AFA*-phycocyanins, notable for their potent antioxidant, anti-inflammatory, and anti-cancer properties, as well as their efficacy in promoting wound healing [14]. Furthermore, this composition encompasses phenylethylamine, a compound recognized for its role as a neuromodulator and its capacity to modulate the immune system [15]. Two important *AFA* extracts, known respectively as AphaMax® and Klamin®, concentrate such molecules, and have shown, in many clinical studies, to produce beneficial effects on a number of diseases.

2. Industrial importance

Circa 120 distinct *AFA* strains have been confirmed globally [12]. However, the strain consumed as a nutritional supplement is found thriving in Klamath Lake, Oregon, USA. This particular strain is identified by its specific name, *Aphanizomenon flos-aquae Ralfs ex Born. & Flah. Var. flos aquae* [7]. Klamath *AFA* nutritional supplements have emerged as a prominent player in the health supplement industry over the past 35 years [7]. Since then, the *AFA* nutritional supplement market is estimated to have reached an overall value of around $100 million a year, indicating a robust consumer interest in *AFA*'s unique benefits [12]. Furthermore, while the majority of Klamath *AFA*'s market is predominantly limited to its use as a nutritional supplement, it is now also expanding into novel areas as well, such as the cosmetic and beauty industry. As the *AFA* industry grows and the availability of its biomass made easier, *AFA*-based products are expected to enter numerous other markets as well, such as the animal feed, aquaculture and biofertiliser ones [12]. The latter holds particular promise because *AFA* stands as the only microalgae or cyanobacterium harvested at scale with the unique capability of nitrogen fixation.

2.1 Harvesting and processing

Klamath *AFA* wild harvesting occurs in Klamath Lake, Oregon, USA, and takes advantage of the unique ecological conditions of this natural habitat (**Figure 2**) [7]. Typically 500–1000 t are harvested per year [12]. The harvesting process is strategically conducted during the *AFA* bloom period, typically occurring in early summer, specifically between the end of June and the beginning of July, and then again in late summer and early fall, between September and November, when environmental factors such as temperature and nutrient availability are optimal [12]. Harvesting begins with the identification of specific areas within the lake where AFA concentrations are high. The desired concentrations range between 5 and 7% solids. Harvesters typically use specialized boats equipped with fine mesh nets or other non-intrusive filtration systems to gently collect the *AFA* from the lake's surface [7].

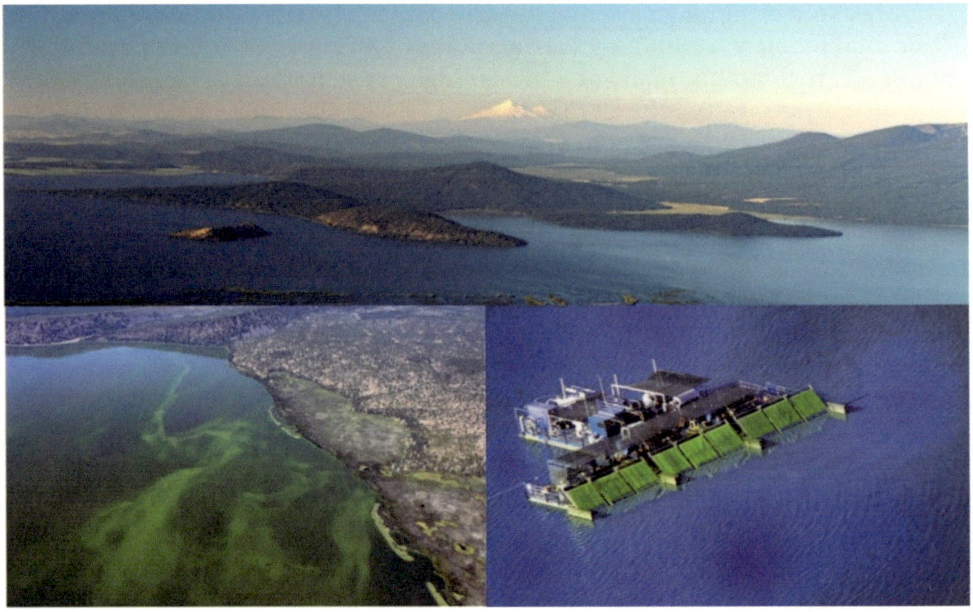

Figure 2.
Klamath Lake, its bloom and the associated harvesting barges. The top image illustrates Klamath Lake with Mount Shasta in the background. The bottom left image is an example of a Klamath AFA bloom, while bottom right of an AFA harvester.

Once harvested, the *AFA* biomass is transported to processing facilities near the lake. In the processing phase, the collected *AFA* undergoes meticulous cleaning processes to remove any impurities or debris, ensuring the purity of the final product. Subsequently, the *AFA* is dewatered in a two-step process: firstly, the majority of the water is removed via a non-specific centrifugation process, and subsequently, it is carefully dried, often utilizing methods like air drying or low temperature drying to preserve its nutritional profile [7]. It is at this moment that the high-value *AFA*-phycocyanin and phenylethylamine compounds are concentrated. High-grade phycocyanin is concentrated through a water-based filtering centrifugation process (Patent: EP2032122A2); while PEA and synergic molecules, such as mycosporine-like aminoacids, are concentrated through water ultrafiltration (Patent: EP2046354B1). The obtained *AFA* biomass and extracts are then commonly transformed into various consumer-friendly forms, such as powders, capsules, or tablets, making it suitable for use as a nutritional supplement [12].

2.2 Wild growth properties

AFA exhibits prolific growth and blooms in Klamath Lake due to a combination of specific ecological factors that create an optimal environment for its thriving population. Klamath Lake measures approximately 52 × 12 km with an approximate surface area of 250 km^2 [16]. Nevertheless, it is a fairly shallow lake, with a mean average depth of 2.4 m. Situated at an altitude of 1300 m, Klamath Lake is bordered by the Cascade Mountains to the west and lies adjacent to a desert area, the Great Basin, to the east [7, 16]. Furthermore, the pristine waters of Klamath Lake are home to a number of different animal species, from the common Sucker fish to Pelicans and Bald Eagles. Currently, the Klamath Basin serves as the primary wintering destination for the most substantial gathering of bald eagles in the contiguous 48 states. Moreover, it functions as the largest rest area for waterfowl along the Pacific flyway [7].

Klamath Lake consistently witnesses numerous *AFA* blooms each year, attributed primarily to its geological origins as a volcanic basin [17]. The lake's geological history traces back 7700 years to the eruption of Mount Mazama, which left substantial mineral sediments at the lake's bottom. Following the explosion, Mount Mazama's crater, now known as Crater Lake, was formed and continues to supply Klamath Lake with water [7]. The mineral-rich composition of Klamath Lake, including elements like Iron, Magnesium, Manganese, Molybdenum, Boron, and Zinc, is a fundamental factor contributing to the formation of *AFA* blooms [18]. These minerals play vital roles in supporting *AFA*'s biological activities; for instance, Molybdenum is crucial for the development and function of the nitrogenase enzyme specific to heterocysts, essential for *AFA*'s nitrogen-fixation capability [19].

The three most important nutrients for *AFA*'s growth, however, are Carbon, Nitrogen and Phosphorous sources [18]. The former is provided by the lake itself due to the occurrence of methane springs across the lake and, of course, of decomposing organic matter. Carbon is expected to compose circa 50% of *AFA*'s total biomass [20]. *AFA*'s consumption of dissolved CO_2 is also reflected in the rise of lake pH from around 7.5 at the start of a bloom to around 9–10 towards the end [18]. CO_2 + water is known to form carbonic acid, thereby lowering the overall pH. Its removal, therefore, leads to the opposite. Nitrogen availability, instead, is not of real concern when it comes to the formation of *AFA* blooms as the cyanobacterium possesses the ability to fix nitrogen directly from the air and convert it into bioavailable forms, like nitrates or nitrites [21]. This ability favors its growth over other organisms, which cannot (see below), allowing it to completely dominate the lake under low-nitrogen conditions [22]. Nevertheless, nitrogen-fixation is costly, from an energetic point of view, and the bioavailability of nitrates/nitrites/ammonia certainly enhances its overall growth rate [23]. The latter nutrient, phosphorous, is most likely the determining factor underlying the amount and frequency of *AFA* blooms, as it would not be able to grow without it. It comes to no surprise that there is an increase in both nitrogen and phosphorous levels in the spring, right before *AFA* starts to bloom [17, 18].

Another critical reason for the formation of *AFA* blooms is that Klamath Lake receives 300 days of sunshine per year, a key factor for the growth of a photosynthetic organism [7]. *AFA* actually possess the capacity to control its buoyancy and height within the water column by generating bubbling vesicles that allow it to float up and down [24]. The consequence is of this is each cell is able to optimize the amount of light needed. Furthermore, Klamath Lake also offers optimal temperatures for *AFA* growth and life cycle. During its blooms, water temperatures will range anywhere between 18 and 25°C [18]. Laboratory studies have found that *AFA*'s optimal growth temperatures for growth range between 20 and 28°C, with a faster growth rate observed between 25 and 28°C [25]. Furthermore, *AFA*'s akinites are able to survive at the lake's sediment during the winter, which can see Upper Klamath Lake freeze over [26].

2.3 Contamination and toxicity

The occurrence of *M. aeruginosa* within the lake has heavily impacted the Klamath *AFA* harvesting business, especially after the government of Oregon introduced the limit of 1 μg of microcystins per gram of cyanobacteria [7].

Microcystins are potent cyclic peptides that, when consumed in elevated quantities, disrupt protein synthesis within liver cells, leading to cellular death and, potentially, organ failure [27]. As a result, Klamath Lake microcystin outbreaks have triggered public health advisories, warning against water contact and consumption. The World Health Organization (WHO) has established a suggested drinking water guideline value of 1 μg/L [28]. Similarly, due to the possible contamination of these toxins within *AFA* blooms, the government of Oregon has imposed an incredibly stringent limit of 1 μg/g of microcystins in Klamath *AFA* supplements [29]. As a result, quality control of *AFA* blooms for microcystin presence has become an important concern. This has not only caused harvesting companies to offhold any *AFA* harvest during the occurrence of *M. aeruginosa*, but has also led to microcystin AFA biomass testing throughout the harvesting and processing stages. This has increased overall costs and any biomass testing higher than 1 μg/g is, for the most part, unusable [12]. Furthermore, microcystin contamination and the associated public concern has also impacted the reputation of *AFA*-based products. Several studies have in fact questioned the safety of *AFA* nutritional supplements, based upon this 1 μg/g requirement [30, 31]. However, there is abundant data to show that the imposed threshold is wrong and should be revisited.

The government of Oregon decided upon this limit by directly translating the WHO limit (1 μg/L) of microcystin in drinking water to Klamath *AFA* biomass. As pointed out by a recent article, there are deep flaws both in this decision, and in the WHO standard [29]. Firstly, the WHO limit is too stringent as it is based upon Fawell et al.'s study which looked at the toxicity (liver damage) of purified microcystins to mice via gavage administration [32]. The methodology employed is not representative of real-world human exposure to these cyanotoxins. Moreover, purified microcystins are not found in nature. Furthermore, the gavage model bypasses the complex interplay between microcystins and the digestive system's protective barriers [29]. While gavage delivers the toxin directly to the gastrointestinal tract, it bypasses the initial enzymatic and acidic breakdown in the stomach, potentially overestimating the bioavailability and subsequent hepatotoxicity observed in real-world scenarios—like that of natural cyanobacterial blooms [29]. Stomach acids and intestinal enzymes inactivate the toxins, almost completely reducing their potency [33]. Unfortunately, most animal studies on microcystin toxicity have been done through the gavage or intraperitoneally injection, and very few reproducing, normal oral ingestion. Studies comparing oral and intraperitoneal administration of microcystins show substantial differences in toxicity [32, 33]. For instance, the other two studies considered by the WHO panel, both of which performed through normal ingestion, generated, for a human being of 60 kg, a safe chronic limit of 45 μg/day and 8.4 μg/day, respectively [34, 35]. The EPA, in fact, recommends, for water consumption, a safety limit of 8 μg/L [36].

This begs for a cautious interpretation of microcystin-related research. Exaggerating the hepatotoxic risks based solely on intravenous studies might create unnecessary public fear and potentially misdirect valuable resources. It is also important to notice that there has been only one animal study investigating the potential toxicity of microcystins within Klamath AFA biomass: mice were administered a diet of *AFA* whole-cell biomass containing 333 μg/g of microcystins over a duration of six months. Subsequent evaluations revealed optimal health conditions, including liver health. The researchers, after implementing all pertinent safety thresholds, deduced that a daily intake of 10 μg/g of microcystins from *AFA* cyanobacterial supplements would be considered safe for an individual weighing 60 kg [28]. Finally and importantly, no human toxicity has ever been reported, even though this biomass has been consumed for decades.

3. Nutraceutical properties

In virtue of its unique ecological setting, wild-harvested Klamath *AFA* emerges as an exceptionally nutrient-dense food source, surpassing many other foods and superfoods in absolute nutritional richness [12]. Its remarkable nutritional profile encompasses all 14 essential vitamins, featuring high concentrations of pro-vitamin A carotenes, substantial levels of B vitamins, crucial for homocysteine regulation, and vitamin K, pivotal for bone health, dental well-being, and blood coagulation [12, 13]. Klamath *AFA* stands out with a mineral content of 73 minerals and trace elements, including noteworthy amounts of iron, natural fluorine, and vanadium, essential for insulin metabolism and addressing metabolic syndrome [12]. Furthermore, it serves as a notable source of Omega-3 fatty acids, with a high quantity of alfa-linoleic acid [13]. It boasts an extensive array of carotenoids, encompassing significant xanthophylls like lutein, canthaxanthin, and lycopene [12]. Recent revelations highlight Klamath *AFA's* richness in polyphenols, featuring a diverse and potent assortment of nutraceutical molecules, including a high quantity of chlorophyll [12, 13, 37]. See **Table 1** for a summary of *AFA's* nutritional profile.

3.1 C-phycocyanin and phycoerythrocyanin

The exceptional anti-inflammatory and antioxidant properties associated with *AFA* and cyanobacteria-based supplements predominantly arise from the intricate composition of pigments, specifically chlorophyll, C-phycocyanin (C-PC), and

Properties	Amount/types	Description
Amino Acids	All 20 amino acids	Essential for life as they are the building blocks of proteins
Protein	~65% of dry mass	Necessary for energy metabolism, all cellular processes and tissue homeostasis
Vitamins	All 14-vitamins: A, K, B1, B3, B5, B9 and B12 are at RDA-relevant amounts	These are necessary nutrients that perform a myriad of essential tasks, from wound healing to bolstering of the immune system
Minerals	All 73 minerals and trace minerals – vanadium, iron, fluoride, iodine, molybdenum, at RDA-relevant amounts	
Chlorophyll	~4% of dry mass	Linked to anti-inflammatory and anti-cancerous effects
Carotenoids	High concentration of canthaxanthin, lutein, and lycopene, plus astaxanthin and zeaxanthin	Lutein possesses eye protection and age-related macular degeneration prevention properties; canthaxanthin is a powerful antioxidant; lycopene is a neuroprotectant
Polyphenols	Caffeic, vanillic and hydroxytyrosol acid	These ameliorate GI tract issues and help prevent the onset of certain metabolic, cardiovascular, and neurodegenerative diseases.
MAA'S	High concentrations of porphyra and shinorine	Linked with antioxidant, immunomodulatory, and anticoagulant activities
PUFA'S	~12–15 mg/g of an omega-3 fatty acid, alfa-linoleic acid (ALA).	ALA reduces the onset likelihood of cardiovascular diseases, IBS, rheumatoid arthritis, and neurodegenerative pathologies. Furthermore, they decrease cholesterol (low-density lipoproteins)
AFA-PC	~60–100 mg/g of biomass	See Section 3.1
PEA	~3 mg/g of biomass	See Section 3.2

Table 1.
Summary of Klamath AFA's nutritional profile.

phycoerythrocyanin (PEC) [38]. Despite comprising around 4% of *AFA*'s total biomass and impacting its taste, chlorophyll proves beneficial in reducing inflammation, aiding in weight loss, and preventing cancer [12, 39]. In the realm of cyanobacteria, *AFA*, much like Spirulina, encompasses both C-phycocyanin (C-PC) and allophycocyanin (AP). Although a 2004 study suggests AFA's phycocyanin content at 15% of the total biomass, recent estimates propose a range of 6–10% [14]. The therapeutic efficacy of C-PC is attributed to their bioactive chromophore, phycocyanobilins (PCB) [40]. Animal studies showcase the effectiveness of C-PC in reducing in vivo edema induced by oxidizing factors and inhibiting liver lipid oxidation caused by hepatotoxic chemicals [41]. As powerful anti-inflammatory agents, C-PC inhibit molecules like NO and, notably, COX-2, serving as selective COX-2 inhibitors without the side effects observed in common NSAIDs [12, 42]. Their reversible antagonism on platelets preserves platelet survival [43]. Furthermore, in-depth in vitro studies validate the potential of C-PC in inhibiting cancer cell proliferation across various tumor cell lines [44]. A comprehensive review affirms their role in cancer treatment, influencing cell cycle arrest, activating apoptotic pathways, and modulating cancer-promoting and fighting molecules [45, 46]. C-PC's diverse effects extend to cardiovascular improvements, wound healing, and immune enhancement, including the normalization of cholesterol levels, platelet aggregation inhibition, cardioprotective roles, fibrinolytic activity, fibroblast release stimulation for wound healing, and immune system support (**Figure 3**) [12, 43].

AFA, unlike *Spirulina*, also expresses the light-harvesting phycoerythrocyanin (PEC) pigment within its phycobilisome. PEC displays a unique chromophore attachment compared to C-PC, one phycoviolobilin (purple color) chromophore

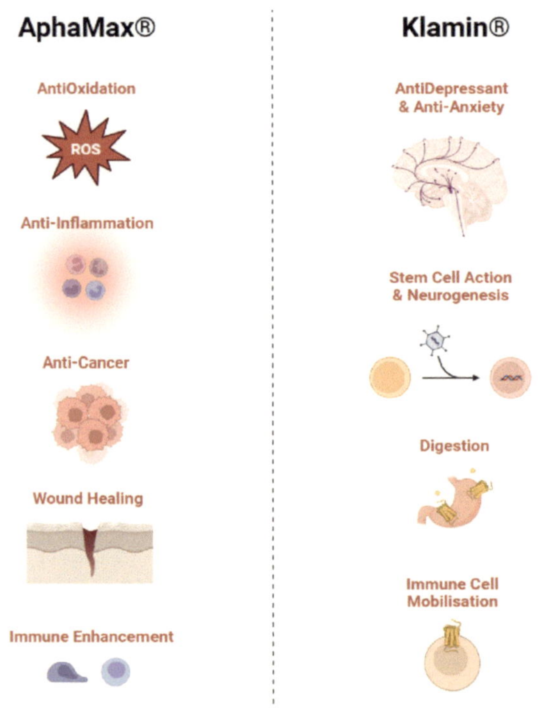

Figure 3.
Summary of AphaMax® and Klamin® nutraceutical properties.

instead of a phycocyanobilin (blue color) [47, 48]. More specifically, both C-PC and PEC are both heterodimeric proteins comprising of monomers that are made of two distinct subunits, α and β. Each αβ monomer typically binds three chromophores. In the case of C-PC each αβ monomer binds three phycocyanobilins, while for PEC it binds two phycocyanobilins and one phycoviolobilin [47–49]. Importantly, the exact nutraceutical properties of phycoviolobilin are yet to be studied. Crucially, the Klamath AFA phycocyanin extract, known as AphaMax®, combines both C-PC and PEC, as the industrial extraction methodology employed cannot discern between the two due to their overall similarity [42]. Recent research has shown that the AFA-phycocyanin extract, AphaMax®, exhibits superior antioxidant and anti-inflammatory responses compared to Spirulina's C-PCs, potentially suggesting that AFA C-PC's activity is enhanced by PEC [12, 14]. For example, in-depth in vitro studies on lipid oxidation showcase AphaMax®'s ability to achieve a 50% inhibition of malonyldialdehyde (MDA), a late by-product of lipid peroxidation, with a dosage 75x lower than *Spirulina*'s PCs (0.14 nM vs. 11.35 μM) and a 90% inhibition 200x lower (1 μM vs. 200 μM) [14]. In terms of inflammation, an unpublished in vitro study on COX-2 enzyme acitivity inhibition, reveals that, at human intake dosages (250 mg), AphaMax® inhibits COX-2 activity by 65%, while *Spirulina* C-PCs by 40%. Overall, there is a clear need to investigate the nutraceutical properties of PEC to better assess the potential nutraceutical impact of AphaMax®.

Numerous other studies have also highlighted AphaMax® anti-inflammatory antioxidation, anti-cancer properties. AphaMax® has the highest oxygen radical absorbance capacity (ORAC) value among all purified molecules, about 300x higher than even quercetin and epigallocatechin [14, 43]. Comparative studies show that while quercetin, at 10 μM, reduces erythrocyte damage by benzoic acid by 25% AphaMax® at 100 nM yields a 95% reduction against copper chloride, a mild oxidative agent like benzoic acid [50]. Furthermore, it should be noted that ORAC tests are limited in their ability to evaluate the full antioxidant spectrum. However, an in vivo human study has demonstrated that long-term AphaMax® administration significantly reduces MDA levels, averaging a 37% reduction within 1–2 months [43]. In terms of cancer, a study testing the efficacy of AphaMax® to inhibit prostate and thyroid cancer cells, showed the ability of the AFA PC & PEC extract to inhibit 95% of cancer cell growth with just 100 nM [51]. In comparison, quercetin and gallic acid only inhibited the proliferation of MCF-7 human breast cancer cells by circa 66% at a concentration of 500 μM, a concentration approximately 5000x higher than the one of AphaMax® [52]. Similarly, at the same concentration of AFA (100 nM), the cannabinoid JWH-33, known for its potent anti-cancer properties, inhibited lung cancer cell proliferation by circa 75%, compared to up to 98% inhibition achieved by AphaMax®. This distinction is significant, as achieving higher levels of inhibition is notably challenging: JWH-33 attains a comparable 95–98% inhibition rate as AFA-PCs, but requires a concentration 1000x higher – 100 μM [53]. In terms of inflammation, a 2006 study investigated effects of AphaMax® in mice. In the experiment, one group of mice received an injection of capsaicin directly into the stomach, leading to a marked increase in inflammation, as measured by Evans Blue extravasation. In a second group, pre-treatment with AFA-PCs extract significantly inhibited inflammation, with an approximate reduction of 95%. A further test involving capsaicin injection in the urinary tract resulted in over 100% inhibition of urinary inflammation [54] (**Figure 4**). This outcome not only demonstrates the potent anti-inflammatory properties of AphaMax® but also their effectiveness at the systemic level after traversing the gastrointestinal tract [54].

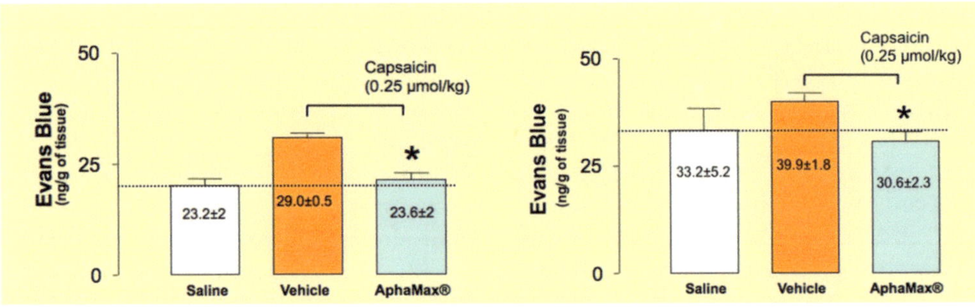

Figure 4.
Bar charts highlighting AphaMax®'s ability (800 mg/kg) to inhibit -induced inflammation as measured by Evans Blue extravasation in mice. Left: Stomach capsaicin injection; right: Urinary bladder capsaicin injection.

AphaMax® has demonstrated also efficacy as a dermatological therapeutic agent in a clinical trial involving human subjects [55]. This study included 10 patients diagnosed with varying stages of psoriasis, who had previously shown no improvement with standard or biologic treatments. Participants were administered three doses of an AphaMax® product daily over a period of three months. Post-treatment assessment revealed substantial remission in 90% of the participants (9 out of 10), with the remaining individual exhibiting significant symptomatic improvement [55]. Additionally, the pharmacological impact of AphaMax® was evaluated in an experimental model of colitis induced by 2,4-dinitrobenzenesulfonic acid (DNBS) in rats [56]. Varied dosages of AphaMax® (20, 50, or 100 mg/kg/day) were administered. The results indicated a notable reduction in histological damage to the colon (**Figure 5**). Furthermore, there was a decrease in myeloperoxidase activity, inhibition of NF-κB activation, and reduced expression of inducible nitric oxide synthase and COX-2. These changes suggest an improvement in the aberrant immune response associated with colonic inflammation. Additionally, the treatment led to a decrease in the inflammatory interleukins IL-1β and IL-6 expression. Finally, AphaMax® exhibited antioxidant properties, evidenced by decreased levels of reactive oxygen species (ROS) and nitrites [56].

3.2 β-Phenylethalamine

A distinguishing feature of AFA is its capacity to produce the endogenous phenolic compound β-phenylethalamine (PEA), setting it apart from other microalgae and cyanobacteria. PEA stands out for its role in neurotransmission, coupled with energizing, anti-anxiety, anti-depressant, and hunger-suppressing properties (**Figure 3**) [12]. This phenolic compound is notably produced during exercise and experiences of "love." It is an agonist to a widely-spread receptor within the body, known as the trace amine-associated receptor (hTAAR) [57]. This is found in the gut, on immune cells and in neuronal synapses. Its activation in the brain, for example, is associated with the release and inhibition of reuptake of biogenic amines such as norepinephrine, dopamine, and serotonin. The resultant increase in catecholamine concentrations can lead to elevated endorphin levels, making PEA an indirect natural painkiller, and an increase in testosterone, contributing to heightened libido. Notably, PEA exhibits rapid and profound effects on mental clarity and alertness without side effects or tolerance [57]. However,

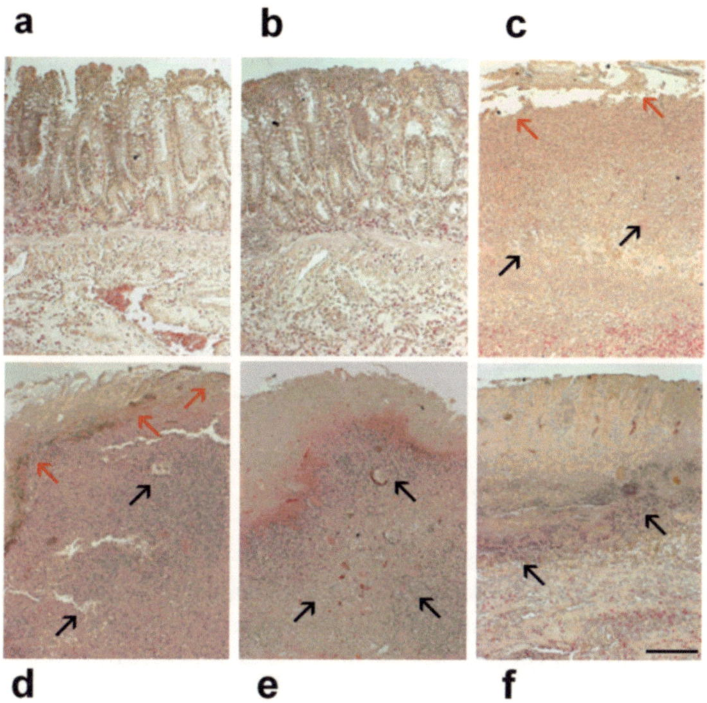

Figure 5.
Effects of Aphamax® on DNBS-induced histological damage in rats. Photomicrographs of the colon stained with hematoxylin & eosin from (a) Sham (control) rats; (b) Sham (control) rats treated with Aphamax® (100 mg/kg); and (c) DNBS rats showing colonic damage and the infiltration of inflammatory cells in mucosa and submucosa. (d), (e), and (f) show DNBS rats treated with Aphamax® at a concentration of 20, 50 and 100 mg/kg, respectively, showing progressive reduction of inflammatory cell infiltration and fewer inflammatory cells close to the mucosal layer. (Scale bar = 100 μm, magnification 20, red arrows = colonic damage, black arrows = inflammatory infiltrate) [56].

the challenge lies in the rapid degradation of purified PEA once ingested: it is a well-known fact that monoamines are rapidly degraded by MAO-B enzymes already in the gut. For this reason, an extract concentrating PEA together with selective MAO-B inhibitors, namely AFA-phycocyanins, Mycosporine-like amino acids (MAAs), and phytochrome C, has been developed. This extract is known as Klamin® [58]. The three molecules are the most potent among all natural substances, and most of all they are reversible inhibitors, blocking the MAO-B activity only temporarily, thus producing no side-effects. This combination facilitates the absorption of a significant portion of PEA through the gut and the blood–brain barrier [15] (**Table 2**).

PEA's crucial attribute lies in its promotion of brain tissue regeneration, as it is able to stimulate the production of erythropoietin (EPO) and its receptor (EPOR). Endogenous erythropoietin (EPO) within the brain acts as a fundamental regulator of neural stem cells, which are totipotent and pivotal for the generation of all neural tissues and neurotransmitters [59]. This positions EPO as a crucial factor in the potential repair and regeneration of brain and nervous system tissues. Notably, the observed changes extend beyond mere functional alterations in EPO dynamics. There is evidence of structural brain changes, notably an increase in EPO receptors [59]. This increase suggests not just a functional modification but also a physical transformation

MAO-B inhibitors	IC_{50}	Ki	Inhibition mode
AFA-phytochrome	0.02	0.01	Mixed
Deprenyl	0.28	0.04	Irreversible
AphaMax®	1.44	0.14	Mixed
AFA MAAs	1.30	0.58	Competitive
Emodin	35.40	15.10	Mixed
Paeonol	42.50	38.20	Competitive
Epicatechine	58.90	21.00	Mixed
Piperine	91.30	79.9	Competitive

IC_{50}: Half-maximal inhibitory concentration; Ki: dissociation constant [15].

Table 2.
Table describing the IC_{50}, Ki and inhibition mode of MAO-B inhibitors concentrated within the Klamin® compared with other synthetic and natural MAO-B inhibitors.

and regeneration of the brain tissues themselves. Such findings hold significant implications for a range of neurodegenerative conditions, including Multiple Sclerosis and Amyotrophic Lateral Sclerosis (ALS). The increased EPO activity and receptor expression could potentially offer new avenues for therapeutic interventions aimed at mitigating the progression of these diseases, emphasizing the role of EPO in neural repair and regeneration mechanisms [12].

One study specifically looked at Klamin® effects on EPO brain levels [58]. Two mice groups, one of group suffering from accelerated senescence (AS) and one not (A), were evaluated on learning ability through the Morris Test (**Figure 6**). After Klamin® administration (100 mg/kg of body weight), the AS mice were able to complete the test 15 s faster than ordinary, from 25 s to 10 s. The normal group of mice (A), instead, lowered the time to complete the test by 4 s, from 9 s to only 5 seconds

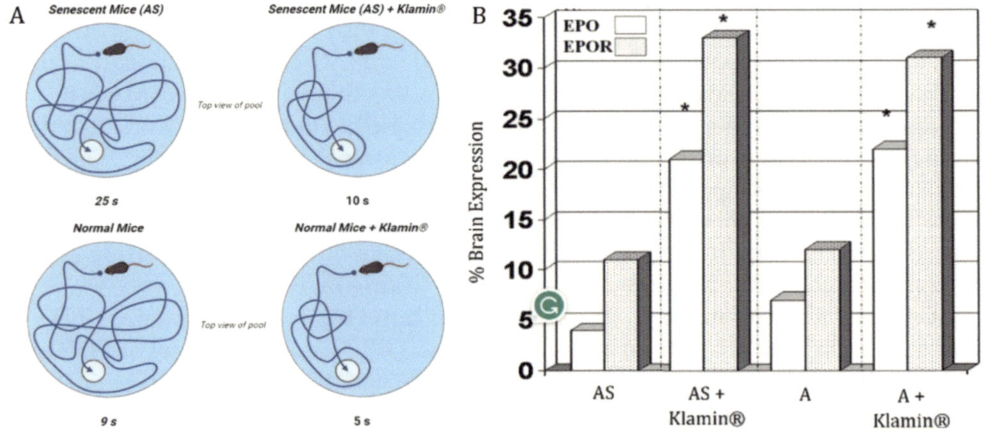

Figure 6.
(A) Illustration of the Morris Water Maze Test, which looks at the learning ability of a mouse to reach the platform (gray circle) and leave the water, and the effect of Klamin® on the mouse speed to reach the platform. (made with biorender). B) Bar chart demonstrating the 500% increase in brain EPO levels and the 300% increase in EPOR following Klamin® administration (100 mg/kg of body weight) in both AS and A mice groups. EPO & EPOR expression were measure via western blot band intensity, with β-actin expression used as the control. Readapted from [58].

[58] (**Figure 6A**). Subsequently, the brain of the mice was analyzed, and the following results were found: a) a strong decrease of brain oxidation (less MDA) and an increase in brain antioxidants (thiols); b) a strong increase in cerebral erythropoietin (EPO) (+500%), as well as in EPO receptors (+300%) [58] (**Figure 6B**). This ability to moderate and mobilize stem cells was already found by a study from Jensen et al., where it was shown that an AFA extract increased the release of stem cells from the bone marrow, triggering the mobilization of CD34+ CD133+ and CD34+ CD133− cells in vivo, associated with repairing of the central nervous system, heart, and other tissues [60].

The AFA PEA extract, due to its ability to increase brain catecholamine levels, has also been investigated for its impact on mental health, including depression, anxiety, ADHD, and autism. Research indicates significant improvements in depression, anxiety, self-esteem, and overall well-being in individuals with depression, including post-menopause and cancer-induced depression [12]. In a study conducted by the Department of Gynecology at the University Hospital of Modena in Italy, a study was carried out involving 40 menopausal women, divided into two groups: 20 receiving Klamin® and 20 in a placebo control group. These participants were selected based on their exhibition of typical psychosomatic symptoms associated with menopause [61]. The intervention group was administered a daily dose of 1 gram of Klamin® for a duration of two months. Post-treatment evaluation using specific psychiatric scales, namely the Kellner-Sheffield Scale and the Zung Self-Rating Scale, revealed a statistically significant improvement in the levels of depression, anxiety, and self-esteem among the women who received Klamin® [61, 62].

Furthermore, Klamin® was also shown to have important beneficial effects on the mood and well-being of terminally ill patients. At the Ovada Oncology Center (Italy), 18 terminally ill cancer patients, being treated only with palliative care, took approximately 1 g of Klamin® for 2 months [63]. Statistically significant improvements were observed in the areas of anxiety, fatigue and depression, confirming that Klamin® is able to balance even apparently conflicting states such as anxiety and depression and to sustain the ability of the body to produce energy [63]. Similarly, Klamin® also had a positive effect on children with ADHD. A recent study looked at 30 children diagnosed with ADHD, and the associated impact of Klamin® administration, at dosages ranging from 0.25–1.20 g (according to weight). The observed improvements were noteworthy, and the areas affected were as follows: 1) the overall condition of the child; 2) the levels of attention and hyperactivity; 3) in executive functions; 4) in the quickness and precision [64]. The researchers also found significant improvements in the 25% of children who were also affected by autistic symptoms [63].

In addition, Klamin® has been shown to have a positive impact on neurodegenerative illnesses, most likely due to its effect on EPO brain levels [12]. Neural stem cell proliferation homeostasis has implications for memory improvement and the reduction of beta-amyloid plaques associated with neurodegenerative diseases, like Alzheimer's. A recent Alzheimer study by Nuzzo et al. demonstrated Klamin®'s ability to prevent the accumulation of the beta-amyloid substance, while inactivating its toxicity [65]. In this study, we administered the oxidizing agent tert-butyl hydroperoxide (TBH) into the mitochondria of live neuronal cells. This intervention resulted in a marked increase in the production of reactive oxygen species (ROS) within the cells, compared to the control group. However, the simultaneous introduction of 0.8 μg of Klamin® alongside TBH effectively inhibited the TBH-induced overproduction of ROS in the mitochondria [65]. Furthermore, the study explored the implications of Klamin® in the context of Alzheimer's disease, particularly its interaction with beta-amyloid, a substance closely associated with the disease's pathogenesis. Human neuronal cultures were stimulated to produce beta-amyloid, and the effect of Klamin® addition was observed. Remarkably, the presence of Klamin® led to a 63% reduction in the production of beta-amyloid compared to the control group [65]. Additionally, the beta-amyloid aggregates that were still formed in the presence of Klamin® were significantly smaller in size and exhibited a substantial loss of toxicity. This result is particularly significant given the role of beta-amyloid aggregates in Alzheimer's disease progression [65].

Klamin®'s nutraceutical properties have also been tested on obesity and its associated metabolic imbalances, which have been linked to neurodegenerative conditions, including Alzheimer's disease. To investigate this connection, a study was conducted on mice using KlamExtra®, a novel product combining Klamin® and Aphamax® extracts [66]. The mice were divided into three groups: one group was fed a standard diet (Lean group), another received a high-fat diet (HFD), and the third group was given a high-fat diet supplemented with the AFA product (HFD + AFA) for a duration of 28 weeks. The study focused on several key aspects: metabolic parameters, brain insulin resistance, the expression of apoptosis (cell death) biomarkers, the modulation of astrocytes and microglia activation markers (key components of brain inflammation), and the accumulation of beta-amyloid plaques, which are characteristic of Alzheimer's disease (**Figure 7**) [66]. These factors were analyzed and compared across the brains of the different mouse groups. Results indicated that the AFA product, KlamExtra®, mitigated neurodegenerative effects induced by the high-fat diet. This included a reduction in insulin resistance and a decrease in neuronal loss. Additionally, AFA supplementation was found to enhance the expression of synaptic proteins and significantly reduce the activation of astrocytes and microglia - a typical response to high-fat diet-induced stress. Moreover, the accumulation of beta-amyloid plaques, often associated with Alzheimer's disease, was also reduced in the mice receiving the AFA supplement [66]. These findings suggest that KlamExtra® has potential therapeutic effects in addressing neurodegeneration linked to obesity and metabolic dysfunctions.

Finally, towards the start of the century, PEA was shown to possess immune enhancement properties. in their 2000 study, Jensen et al. discovered that consuming 1.5 g of AFA biomass leads to a broad enhancement of immune surveillance, without directly stimulating the immune system [67]. This enhancement is characterized by a rapid increase in the movement of immune cells, such as monocytes and lymphocytes, from bodily tissues into the bloodstream. Specifically, there is a notable

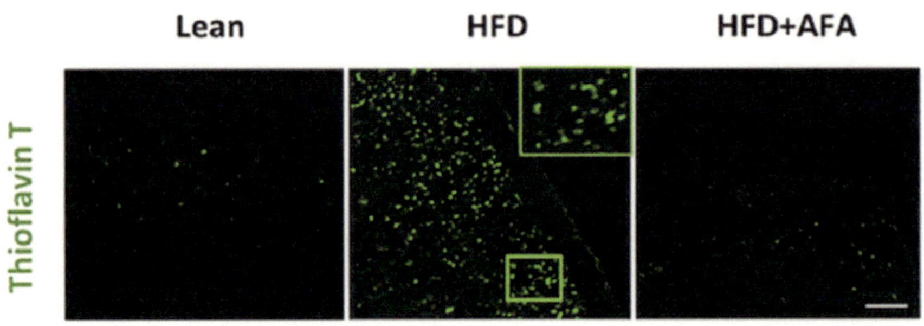

Figure 7.
Thioflavin T staining of beta-amyloid aggregates on cerebral cortex section of lean, HFD and HFD + AFA mice. Thioflavin T-positive amyloid deposits are prominent in cortex areas of HFD mouse compared with those from lean and HFD + AFA.

mobilization of CD3+, CD4+, CD8+ T cells, and CD19+ B cells. Notably, individuals who regularly consume AFA biomass exhibit a 40% increase in natural killer (NK) cell recruitment within 4–6 hours post-ingestion [67]. The study attributes this immune modulation to various low-molecular compounds present in the AFA cyanobacteria, with PEA likely being a key contributor. PEA acts as an agonist to TAAR, which are found on monocytes, B cells, T cells, and NK cells. The stimulation of these cells by PEA is thought to be a crucial factor in their mobilization and the resultant enhanced immune surveillance observed following AFA biomass ingestion [68].

4. Conclusion

AFA, sourced from Klamath Lake, Oregon, is an example of nutritional excellence and industrial relevance in the health supplement sector. This wild-harvested cyanobacterium, flourishing in the lake's unique volcanic ecosystem, boasts a rich nutritional profile, ranging from a high protein content, up to 70%, to an elevated concentration of Omega-3 s PUFAs. The nutraceutical value of AFA is epitomized by its specialized extracts, AphaMax® and Klamin®. AphaMax® is enriched with C-PC and PEC and confers notable anti-inflammatory benefits, due to its ability to reversibly inhibit the inflammatory COX-2 enzyme, while also having important antioxidant, anti-cancer and dermatological properties. On the other hand, Klamin®, containing β-phenylethylamine (PEA), has shown significant potential in improving mental health. It is particularly effective in alleviating symptoms of depression and anxiety, as shown in post-menopausal women and cancer patients, due to PEA's ability to increase brain catecholamine concentrations. Additionally, its promising results in managing ADHD and its potential in treating neurodegenerative diseases such as Alzheimer's further underscore its therapeutic versatility. In conclusion, AFA from Klamath Lake emerges as a powerhouse of health benefits, especially through its extracts AphaMax® and Klamin®. Its impressive nutritional profile and the health-promoting properties of its extracts solidify its standing as an invaluable component in the realm of nutritional supplements.

Conflict of interest

Scoglio, S. & Scoglio G. D. own and manage a Klamath AFA harvesting and nutritional supplement company.

Author details

Stefano Scoglio[1*] and Gabriel Dylan Scoglio[2]

1 Centro di Ricerche Nutriterapiche, Urbino, Italy

2 Department of Structural and Molecular Biology, University College London, London, UK

*Address all correspondence to: stefanoscoglio@me.com

References

[1] Mehdizadeh Allaf M, Peerhossaini H. Cyanobacteria: Model microorganisms and beyond. Microorganisms. 2022;**10**(4):696

[2] Rasmussen B, Fletcher IR, Brocks JJ, Kilburn MR. Reassessing the first appearance of eukaryotes and cyanobacteria. Nature. 2008;**455**(7216):1101-1104

[3] Whitton BA, Potts M. Introduction to the cyanobacteria. Ecology of cyanobacteria II: Their Diversity in Space and Time. Dodrecht: Springer; 2012. pp. 1-13

[4] Arias DM, Ortíz-Sánchez E, Okoye PU, Rodríguez-Rangel H, Ortega AB, Longoria A, et al. A review on cyanobacteria cultivation for carbohydrate-based biofuels: Cultivation aspects, polysaccharides accumulation strategies, and biofuels production scenarios. Science of The Total Environment. 2021;**794**:148636

[5] Cuellar-Bermudez SP, Aleman-Nava GS, Chandra R, Garcia-Perez JS, Contreras-Angulo JR, Markou G, et al. Nutrients utilization and contaminants removal. A review of two approaches of algae and cyanobacteria in wastewater. Algal Research. 2017;**24**:438-449

[6] Soni RA, Sudhakar K, Rana R. Spirulina–From growth to nutritional product: A review. Trends in Food Science & Technology. 2017;**69**:157-171

[7] Carmichael WW, Drapeau C, Anderson DM. Harvesting of Aphanizomenon flos-aquae Ralfs ex Born. & Flah. var. flos-aquae (Cyanobacteria) from Klamath Lake for human dietary use. Journal of Applied Phycology. 2000;**12**:585-595

[8] Cirés S, Ballot A. A review of the phylogeny, ecology and toxin production of bloom-forming Aphanizomenon spp. and related species within the Nostocales (cyanobacteria). Harmful Algae. 2016;**54**:21-43

[9] Grewe CB, Pulz O. The Biotechnology of cyanobacteria. Ecology of cyanobacteria II: Their Diversity in Space and Time. Dodrecht: Springer; 2012. pp. 707-739

[10] Kumar K, Mella-Herrera RA, Golden JW. Cyanobacterial heterocysts. Cold Spring Harbor Perspectives in Biology. 2010;**2**(4):a000315

[11] Kaplan-Levy RN, Hadas O, Summers ML, Rücker J, Sukenik A. Akinetes: Dormant cells of cyanobacteria. Dormancy and Resistance in Harsh Environments. In: Topics in Current Genetics. Vol. 21. Berlin, Heidelberg: Springer; 2010. pp. 5-27

[12] Scoglio GD, Jackson H, Purton S. The commercial potential of Aphanizomenon flos-aquae, a nitrogen-fixing edible cyanobacterium. The Journal of Applied Phycology. 2023

[13] Sandgruber F, Gielsdorf A, Baur AC, Schenz B, Müller SM, Schwerdtle T, et al. Variability in macro-and micronutrients of 15 commercially available microalgae powders. Marine Drugs. 2021;**19**(6):310

[14] Benedetti S, Benvenuti F, Pagliarani S, Francogli S, Scoglio S, Canestrari F. Antioxidant properties of a novel phycocyanin extract from the blue-green alga Aphanizomenon flos-aquae. Life Sciences. 2004;**75**(19):2353-2362

[15] Scoglio S, Benedetti Y, Benvenuti F, Battistelli S, Canestrari F, Benedetti S.

Selective monoamine oxidase B inhibition by an Aphanizomenon flos-aquae extract and by its constitutive active principles phycocyanin and mycosporine-like amino acids. Phytomedicine. 2014;**21**(7):992-997

[16] Walker W, Walker J, Kann J. Evaluation of water and nutrient balances for the Upper Klamath Lake Basin in water years 1992-2010. Prepared for Klamath Tribes Natural Resources Department, Chiloquin, Oregon by Environmental Engineers, Concord, Massachusetts and Aquatic Ecosystem Sciences, Ashland, Oregon. 2012;50

[17] Essaid HI, Kuwabara JS, Corson-Dosch NT, Carter JL, Topping BR. Evaluating the dynamics of groundwater, lakebed transport, nutrient inflow and algal blooms in upper Klamath Lake, Oregon, USA. Science of The Total Environment. 2021;**765**:142768

[18] Eldridge SLC, Wood TM, Echols KR. Spatial and temporal dynamics of cyanotoxins and their relation to other water quality variables in upper Klamath Lake, Oregon, 2007-09: US Department of the Interior, US Geological Survey; 2012

[19] Seefeldt LC, Hoffman BM, Dean DR. Mechanism of Mo-dependent nitrogenase. Annual Review of Biochemistry. 2009;**78**:701-722

[20] Huang Y, Li P, Chen G, Peng L, Chen X. The production of cyanobacterial carbon under nitrogen-limited cultivation and its potential for nitrate removal. Chemosphere. 2018;**190**:1-8

[21] Berman T. The role of DON and the effect of N: P ratios on occurrence of cyanobacterial blooms: Implications from the outgrowth of Aphanizomenon in Lake Kinneret. Limnology and Oceanography. 2001;**46**(2):443-447

[22] Latysheva N, Junker VL, Palmer WJ, Codd GA, Barker D. The evolution of nitrogen fixation in cyanobacteria. Bioinformatics. 2012;**28**(5):603-606

[23] Mansouri H, Talebizadeh B, Salajegheh Ansari MM. Study on the effect of sodium nitroprusside on growth and nitrogen fixation in blue-green algae nostoc linckia. Iranian Journal of Science and Technology, Transactions A: Science. 2019;**43**:2083-2090

[24] Porat R, Teltsch B, Perelman A, Dubinsky Z. Diel buoyancy changes by the cyanobacterium Aphanizomenon ovalisporum from a shallow reservoir. Journal of Plankton Research. 2001;**23**(7):753-763

[25] Debella HJ. Mass culture of Aphanizomenon flos-aquae Ralfs EX Born and Flah var. flos-aquae (cyanobacteria) from Klamath Falls, Oregon, USA, in closed chamber bioreactors. Ethiop Journal of Biological Sciences. 2005;**4**(2):135-145

[26] Yamamoto Y, Nakahara H. Life cycle of cyanobacterium Aphanizomenon flos-aquae. Taiwania. 2009;54(2):113-117

[27] Rastogi RP, Sinha RP, Incharoensakdi A. The cyanotoxin-microcystins: Current overview. Reviews in Environmental Science and Bio/Technology. 2014;**13**:215-249

[28] Schaeffer DJ, Malpas PB, Barton LL. Risk assessment of microcystin in dietary Aphanizomenon flos-aquae. Ecotoxicology and Environmental Safety. 1999;**44**(1):73-80

[29] Scoglio S. Microcystins in water and in microalgae: Do microcystins as microalgae contaminants warrant the current public alarm? Toxicology Reports. 2018;**5**:785-792

[30] Lyon-Colbert A, Su S, Cude C. A systematic literature review for evidence of Aphanizomenon flos-aquae toxigenicity in recreational waters and toxicity of dietary supplements: 2000-2017. Toxins. 2018;**10**(7):254

[31] Saker ML, Jungblut A-D, Neilan BA, Rawn DF, Vasconcelos VM. Detection of microcystin synthetase genes in health food supplements containing the freshwater cyanobacterium Aphanizomenon flos-aquae. Toxicon. 2005;**46**(5):555-562

[32] Fawell J, Mitchell R, Everett D, Hill R. The toxicity of cyanobacterial toxins in the mouse: I microcystin-LR. Human & Experimental Toxicology. 1999;**18**(3):162-167

[33] Moreno IM, Maraver J, Aguete EC, Leao M, Gago-Martínez A, Cameán AM. Decomposition of microcystin-LR, microcystin-RR, and microcystin-YR in water samples submitted to in vitro dissolution tests. Journal of Agricultural and Food Chemistry. 2004;**52**(19):5933-5938

[34] Falconer IR, Smith JV, Jackson AR, Jones A, Runnegar MT. Oral toxicity of a bloom of the cyanobacterium Microcystis aeruginosa administered to mice over periods up to 1 year. Journal of Toxicology and Environmental Health, Part A Current Issues. 1988;**24**(3):291-305

[35] Falconer IR, Burch MD, Steffensen DA, Choice M, Coverdale OR. Toxicity of the blue-green alga (cyanobacterium) Microcystis aeruginosa in drinking water to growing pigs, as an animal model for human injury and risk assessment. Environmental Toxicology and Water Quality. 1994;**9**(2):131-139

[36] (EPA) USEPA. Recommended human health recreational ambient water quality criteria or swimming advisories for Microcystins and Cylindrospermopsin. 2019:1-249

[37] Righi V, Parenti F, Schenetti L, Mucci A. Mycosporine-like amino acids and other phytochemicals directly detected by high-resolution NMR on Klamath (Aphanizomenon flos-aquae) blue-green algae. Journal of Agricultural and Food Chemistry. 2016;**64**(35):6708-6715

[38] Saini DK, Pabbi S, Shukla P. Cyanobacterial pigments: Perspectives and biotechnological approaches. Food and Chemical Toxicology. 2018;**120**:616-624

[39] Koyande AK, Chew KW, Rambabu K, Tao Y, Chu D-T, Show P-L. Microalgae: A potential alternative to health supplementation for humans. Food Science and Human Wellness. 2019;**8**(1):16-24

[40] Manirafasha E, Ndikubwimana T, Zeng X, Lu Y, Jing K. Phycobiliprotein: Potential microalgae derived pharmaceutical and biological reagent. Biochemical Engineering Journal. 2016;**109**:282-296

[41] Romay C, Gonzalez R, Ledon N, Remirez D, Rimbau V. C-phycocyanin: A biliprotein with antioxidant, anti-inflammatory and neuroprotective effects. Current Protein and Peptide Science. 2003;**4**(3):207-216

[42] Benedetti S, Rinalducci S, Benvenuti F, Francogli S, Pagliarani S, Giorgi L, et al. Purification and characterization of phycocyanin from the blue-green alga Aphanizomenon flos-aquae. Journal of Chromatography B. 2006;**833**(1):12-18

[43] Benedetti S, Benvenuti F, Scoglio S, Canestrari F. Oxygen radical

absorbance capacity of phycocyanin and phycocyanobilin from the food supplement Aphanizomenon flos-aquae. Journal of Medicinal Food. 2010;**13**(1):223-227

[44] Li B, Chu X, Gao M, Li W. Apoptotic mechanism of MCF-7 breast cells in vivo and in vitro induced by photodynamic therapy with C-phycocyanin. Acta Biochimica et Biophysica Sinica. 2009;**42**(1):80-89

[45] Jiang L, Wang Y, Yin Q, Liu G, Liu H, Huang Y, et al. Phycocyanin: A potential drug for cancer treatment. Journal of Cancer. 2017;**8**(17):3416-3429

[46] Braune S, Krüger-Genge A, Kammerer S, Jung F, Küpper J-H. Phycocyanin from Arthrospira platensis as potential anti-cancer drug: Review of In vitro and In vivo studies. Life. 2021;**11**(2):91

[47] MacColl R. Cyanobacterial phycobilisomes. Journal of Structural Biology. 1998;**124**(2):311-334

[48] Stadnichuk IN, Krasilnikov PM, Zlenko DV. Cyanobacterial phycobilisomes and phycobiliproteins. Microbiology. 2015;**84**(2):101-111

[49] Basheva D, Moten D, Stoyanov P, Belkinova D, Mladenov R, Teneva I. Content of phycoerythrin, phycocyanin, alophycocyanin and phycoerythrocyanin in some cyanobacterial strains: Applications. Engineering in Life Sciences. 2018;**18**(11):861-866

[50] Baş H, Kalender S, Pandir D. In vitro effects of quercetin on oxidative stress mediated in human erythrocytes by benzoic acid and citric acid. Folia Biologica. 2014;**62**(1):57-64

[51] Scoglio S, Lo Curcio V, Catalani S, Palma F, Battistelli S, Benedetti S. Inhibitory effects of Aphanizomenon flos-aquae constituents on human UDP-glucose dehydrogenase activity. Journal of Enzyme Inhibition and Medicinal Chemistry. 2016;**31**(6):1492-1497

[52] Hwang EY, Huh J-W, Choi M-M, Choi SY, Hong H-N, Cho S-W. Inhibitory effects of gallic acid and quercetin on UDP-glucose dehydrogenase activity. FEBS Letters. 2008;**582**(27):3793-3797

[53] Vidinský B, Gál P, Pilátová M, Vidová Z, Solár P, Varinská L, et al. Anti-proliferative and anti-angiogenic effects of CB2R agonist (JWH-133) in non-small lung cancer cells (A549) and human umbilical vein endothelial cells: An in vitro investigation. Folia Biologica. 2012;**58**(2):75-80

[54] Kuriakose GC, Kurup MG. Evaluation of renoprotective effect of Aphanizomenon flos-aquae on cisplatin-induced renal dysfunction in rats. Renal Failure. 2008;**30**(7):717-725

[55] Cavalchini A, Scoglio S. Complementary treatment of psoriasis with an AFA-phycocyanins product: A preliminary 10-cases study. International Medical Journal. 2009;**16**:221-224

[56] Zizzo MG, Caldara G, Bellanca A, Nuzzo D, Di Carlo M, Scoglio S, et al. AphaMax(®), an Aphanizomenon flos-aquae aqueous extract, exerts intestinal protective effects in experimental colitis in rats. Nutrients. 2020;**12**(12)

[57] Irsfeld M, Spadafore M, Prüß BM. β-Phenylethylamine, a small molecule with a large impact. Webmedcentral. 2013;**4**(9):4409

[58] Sedriep S, Xia X, Marotta F, Zhou L, Yadav H, Yang H, et al. Beneficial nutraceutical modulation of cerebral erythropoietin expression and oxidative stress: An experimental study. Journal of

Biological Regulators and Homeostatic Agents. 2011;**25**(2):187-194

[59] Noguchi CT, Asavaritikrai P, Teng R, Jia Y. Role of erythropoietin in the brain. Critical Reviews in Oncology/Hematology. 2007;**64**(2):159-171

[60] Jensen GS, Hart AN, Zaske LAM, Drapeau C, Gupta N, Schaeffer DJ, et al. Mobilization of human CD34+CD133+ and CD34+CD133− stem cells in vivo by consumption of an extract from Aphanizomenon flos-aquae—Related to modulation of CXCR4 expression by an L-selectin ligand? Cardiovascular Revascularization Medicine. 2007;**8**(3):189-202

[61] Genazzani AD, Chierchia E, Lanzoni C, Santagni S, Veltri F, Ricchieri F, et al. Effects of Klamath algae extract on psychological disorders and depression in menopausal women: A pilot study. Minerva Ginecologica. 2010;**62**(5):381-388

[62] Scoglio S, Benedetti S, Canino C, Santagni S, Rattighieri E, Chierchia E, et al. Effect of a 2-month treatment with Klamin, a Klamath algae extract, on the general well-being, antioxidant profile and oxidative status of postmenopausal women. Gynecological Endocrinology. 2009;**25**(4):235-240

[63] Bellingeri P, Bonucci M, Scoglio S. Complementary treatment of mood disturbances in terminally ill oncological patients with the Aphanizomenon flos aquae extract Klamin®. Advances in Complementary and Alternative Medicine. 2018;**1**:1-5

[64] Cremonte M, Sisti D, Maraucci I, Giribone S, Colombo E, Rocchi MBL, et al. The effect of experimental supplementation with the Klamath algae extract Klamin on attention-deficit/hyperactivity disorder. Journal of Medicinal Food. 2017;**20**(12):1233-1239

[65] Nuzzo D, Presti G, Picone P, Galizzi G, Gulotta E, Giuliano S, et al. Effects of the Aphanizomenon flos-aquae extract (Klamin®) on a neurodegeneration cellular model. Oxidative Medicine and Cellular Longevity. 2018;**2018**:9089016

[66] Galizzi G, Deidda I, Amato A, Calvi P, Terzo S, Caruana L, et al. Aphanizomenon flos-aquae (AFA) extract prevents neurodegeneration in the HFD mouse model by modulating astrocytes and microglia activation. International Journal of Molecular Sciences. 2023;**24**(5):9089016

[67] Jensen GS, Ginsberg DI, Huerta P, Citton M, Drapeau C. Consumption of Aphanizomenon flos-aquae has rapid effects on the circulation and function of immune cells in humans. Journal of the American Nutraceutical Association. 2000;**2**:50-58

[68] Babusyte A, Kotthoff M, Fiedler J, Krautwurst D. Biogenic amines activate blood leukocytes via trace amine-associated receptors TAAR1 and TAAR2. Journal of Leukocyte Biology. 2013;**93**(3):387-394

Chapter 5

Cyanobacteria: A Promising Future for Sustainable Agriculture

Seyed Mojtaba Soleymani Robati

Abstract

Cyanobacteria are photosynthetic prokaryotes that can be considered as a promising source for environment-friendly sustainable agriculture. Various species of cyanobacteria have been described as biofertilizers and plant biostimulants. They can affect nutrient utilization efficiency, plant growth, gene expression, and the quality and quantity characteristics of the phytochemical composition of plants by producing many highly effective chemical compounds such as enzymes and hormones. Cyanobacteria can also induce plant resistance against biotic and non-biotic stresses. They increase plant tolerance through their direct effect on the soil or by induction of activation of plant reactions. Cyanobacteria can reduce the effect of salinity by producing extracellular polysaccharides or compatible solutions, and increase germination in drought conditions. Cyanobacteria activate plant defense responses to control plant pathogens as the inducer of systemic plant resistance against pathogens, and also, they are an effective strategy as a biocide against bacteria, fungi, and nematodes that attack plants.

Keywords: cyanobacteria, sustainable agriculture, biostimulants, biofertilizer, bioactive compound, phytohormones

1. Introduction

Conventional agriculture involves large-scale use of synthetic fertilizers, and pesticides to increase food production and address the needs of a rapidly growing population. However, this approach has hurt soil microbes, resulting in a reduction of agricultural output. As an alternative, sustainable agriculture focuses on addressing societal concerns about food quality and environmental protection through better management practices. One such practice is using microbial fertilizers as plant growth promoters to improve yields. Cyanobacteria are a type of plant growth-promoting microbes (PGPMs) that are commonly used in sustainable agriculture [1, 2]. These prokaryotic photoautotrophic microorganisms, some of which are facultative heterotrophs, can thrive in various environments, even in extreme conditions [3]. Cyanobacteria can be biofertilizers to solubilize phosphate, improve soil structure and nutrient uptake, and reduce soil salinity. They are also capable of increasing soil nitrogen content through nitrogen fixation from the atmosphere, making them a valuable addition to biofertilizers [4]. Additionally, cyanobacteria produce bioactive molecules like phytohormones, polysaccharides, phenolic compounds, and amino acids that can serve as high-quality biostimulants, promoting plant growth and improving physiological functions. These metabolites also play a vital role in protecting plants against abiotic stresses and helping them fight against pests and pathogens.

2. Cyanobacterial biofertilizer

Cyanobacteria are one of the most important groups of microorganisms that are used as biofertilizers in sustainable agriculture. The common reasons for using cyanobacteria as biofertilizers are their ability for nitrogen fixation, soil amendment, and solubilization of phosphate in the soil.

2.1 Nitrogen fixation by cyanobacteria

In intensive agriculture, nitrogen (N) supplementation is done through the application of N-rich fertilizers such as urea and ammonium sulfate to the soil. However, 50% of nitrogen is lost to the environment due to ammonia volatilization, denitrification, leaching, and surface runoff, and only 50% of N is absorbed by the plant, and this is the major drawback of the mentioned method. To solve this problem, the lack of soil nitrogen content can be corrected by fixing atmospheric nitrogen. Atmospheric nitrogen (N_2), the most abundant source of nitrogen in the earth, is very stable because of the triple bond between the nitrogen atoms; almost inert N_2 can be chemically reduced to NH_3, but it is only possible at very high temperatures and high pressures of N_2 and H_2 (Haber-Bosch process). Therefore, in order to increase uptake by plants, this process requires high energy to reduce N_2 to ammonia [5, 6].

Atmospheric nitrogen fixation is one of the most important functions of cyanobacteria, which are used as biofertilizers. As the main nitrogen-fixing agents in agricultural soils, they fix atmospheric nitrogen and are then re-assimilated by higher plants [6, 7]. Importantly, cyanobacteria fix N_2 at ambient pressure and temperature; however, it is still an energetically expensive process for N_2-fixing organisms. Nitrogenase requires 16 ATP and 8 low potential electrons to reduce N_2 to NH_3 (usually provided as reduced ferredoxin) [5]. Nitrogenase is inactivated by oxygen, so oxygenic photosynthesis and nitrogen fixation processes are incompatible [8].

To solve the problem, two different mechanisms have evolved to separate two processes: First process is temporal separation (day-night rhythm): Nitrogen, accumulated during the day by stored glycogen granules in the form of a nitrogen-rich polymer (cyanophycin), is fixed at night [9, 10]. Another process is spatial separation (cell differentiation). Some cyanobacteria, such as *Anabaena*, are able to fix nitrogen during the day with the help of specialized cells the so-called heterocysts. Because heterocysts do not have photosystem II and do not fix carbon, photosynthesis does not occur in them; as a result, nitrogenase is not inactivated by oxygen [5, 11].

Heterocyst-based N_2 fixation is the most dominant and common mechanism in cyanobacteria. This process can occur as a symbiotic relationship between cyanobacterial species and the host plant in which the microorganisms colonize the leaves and roots of the host plant [12]. In plant leaves, cyanobacteria first enter the tissue through the stomata and then colonize the intercellular spaces by forming a cyanobacterial ring; while in the roots, loose and strong colonies are formed on root hairs and root surfaces, respectively [6, 13]. Larger and rounder shapes, thicker cell walls,

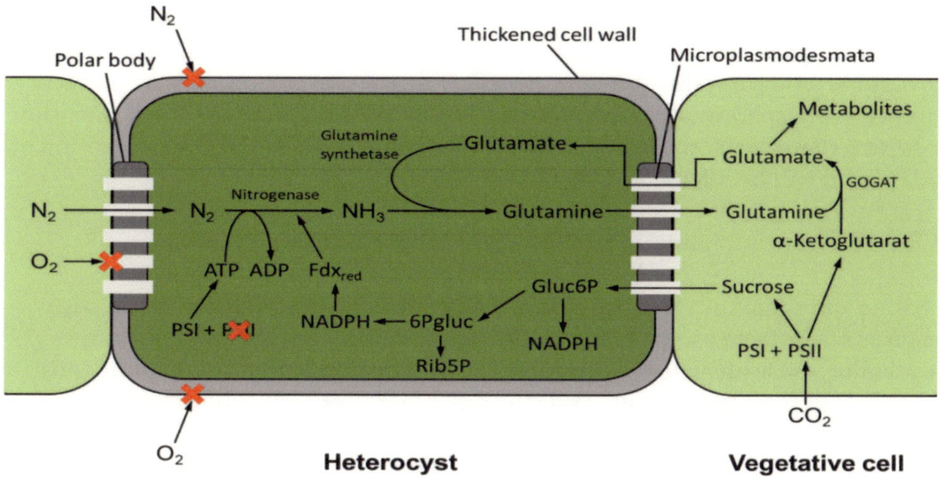

Figure 1.
Nitrogen fixation process and metabolic exchange between heterocysts and neighboring vegetative cells. 6Pgluc = gluconate-6-phosphate, Gluc6P = glucose-6-phosphate, Rib5P = ribulose-5-phosphate, PSI = photosystem I, PSII = photosystem II, Fdxred = reduced ferredoxin, and GOGAT = glutamate synthase [10].

and accumulation of cyanophycin granules at the border with neighboring cells distinguish heterocysts from vegetative cells [10, 14]. The schematic of nitrogen fixation in heterocysts of cyanobacteria is shown in **Figure 1**.

2.2 Phosphorus uptake by cyanobacteria

Phosphorus, as an essential mineral for plant growth and development, is the limiting nutrient for biomass production in agriculture, its availability in the highest amount (after nitrogen) is required for plant growth and yield, and it plays a key role in storing and using energy by soil microorganisms. However, plants or microbes are likely to be challenged to obtain phosphorus from the soil in order to grow, because a large part of soil organic phosphorus becomes inaccessible through fixation or adsorption to clay soil particles [15] and also, phosphorus is forced into relatively inaccessible inorganic pools as a result of mineral phase precipitation reactions with calcium and magnesium in alkaline soils, and iron and aluminum in acidic soils. Therefore, phosphate fertilizers are often added to the soil [16].

To release phosphate from inorganic and organic pools of total soil phosphorus, cyanobacteria, as specific phosphate-solubilizing microorganisms, are used [17]. Cyanobacteria probably solubilize phosphate by two mechanisms. First is the release of organic acids which can solubilize phosphorus [18], and the second mechanism is to synthesize a calcium ions (Ca^{2+}) chelator which directs the dissolution in the correct direction without changing the pH of the growth medium [19]. The important role of cyanobacteria in mobilization of inorganic phosphates is performed through extracellular phosphatases; by extracting the organic acids enzymatic profile of the soil inoculated with cyanobacteria, it was found that acid phosphatases and alkaline phosphatases are involved in phosphate solubilization, so inoculating soils with species such as *Nostoc* and *Anabaena* is promising [18, 19]. Less-soluble phosphorus forms like calcium phosphate [$Ca_3(PO_4)_2$], ferric phosphate ($FePO_4$), aluminum phosphate ($AlPO_4$), and hydroxyapatite [($Ca_5(PO_4)_3.OH$)] in soil, sediments, or pure culture can be solubilized by cyanobacteria, improving the bioavailability of phosphorus to the plants [20]. Besides the above-mentioned two mechanisms, there is also a third possibility. At this mechanism, available phosphorus could be removed by cyanobacteria from the sphere of chemical fixation in soil by absorbing excess amounts of phosphorous or incorporating it into cell constituents for cell nutrition needs, and then over some time (through exudation or microbial decomposition of dead cells) it will be released gradually to the plants [21].

2.3 The role of cyanobacteria in saline and sodic soil amendment

Saline and sodic soils that are rich in salt and/or have an alkaline nature, also known as salt-affected soils, are typically not conducive to the growth of plants [22]. The alkaline soil is identified by its high pH, plentiful exchangeable sodium ions, elevated electrical conductivity, and substantial presence of carbonates [23]. This type of soil has restricted aeration, inadequate hydraulic conductivity, and elevated osmotic pressure, hindering plant roots and absorption of water and nutrients. The high salinity of the soil, due to increased osmotic stress and build-up of sodium and chloride ions, can negatively affect plants' metabolic activities and growth. Moreover, salt stress can diminish the microbial population in the soil and affect carbon cycling. The high concentration of salt in these soils leads to the formation of a rugged and water-resistant layer [22, 24–26].

Cyanobacteria, in association with plants, play a crucial role in mitigating salt stress. The effective use of cyanobacteria in the remediation of agricultural soils affected by salt has been proven across a variety of soil types and weather conditions [27]. Numerous species of cyanobacteria have the ability to adapt to different salinity conditions. Cyanobacteria in the rhizosphere instigate salt tolerance in crops and protect them from salt disruption. Many studies show the enhancements in the growth and yield of key crops like wheat, maize, and rice, credited to the direct de-salinization by cyanobacteria [27, 28]. Cyanobacteria through various mechanisms improve saline and sodic soils. These encompass active ion expulsion, nitrogen fixation, synthesis of phytohormones, supply of compatible solutes, discharge of extracellular polymeric substances, and a variety of defense enzymes during the process of soil reclamation [28–30]. Cyanobacteria can increase the soil's water retention and biomass after their death and decomposition [31]. Furthermore, some cyanobacterial species can eliminate soluble sodium from the soil *via* a process known as biosorption. The amendment of soil structure by cyanobacteria, especially the creation of soil channels, aids in the relocation of salt to deeper soil layers, thus minimizing damage to crops. The cyanobacterial extracellular polymeric have the ability to bind sodium ions and create biofilms, thereby safeguarding plants from salt-induced stress [27, 32].

3. Cyanobacterial biostimulant

Biostimulants are a distinct compound from biofertilizer that has a direct effect on plants regardless of nutrient content, increasing crop productivity. By applying plant biostimulants on plants, natural mechanisms related to increasing plant growth, nutrient utilization efficiency, and tolerance to abiotic stress factors are stimulated [33, 34]. In the scientific community, cyanobacteria and microalgae are known as promising biological sources for the production of a new class of high-quality biostimulants, which is why today the main focus is on these microorganisms. Cyanobacteria are able to produce bioactive molecules, affecting plants even at low

DOI: http://dx.doi.org/10.5772/intechopen.1005021

Class	Metabolites	Cyanobacterial strains
Phytohormones	Auxins, abscisic acid, cytokinins, gibberellins, ethylene	*Anabaena* sp., *Oscillatoria* sp., *Nostoc* sp., *Phormidium* sp., *Scytonema* sp., *Synechocystis* sp., and *Westiellopsis prolifica*
Phenolic compounds	Flavonoids, phenolic acids, cell wall phenolics	*Arthrospira* sp., *Anabaena* sp., *Calothrix*, *Oscillatoria*, *Chroococcidiopsis*, *Nostoc* sp., *Leptolyngbya*, *Phormidium*.
Terpenoids	Isoprene, limonene, linalool, β-phellandrene, farnesene, bisabolene	*Anabaena* sp., *Synechococcus* sp., *Synechocystis* sp.
Carotenoids	β-Carotene, astaxanthin, zeaxanthin, canthaxanthin, lutein, lycopene, echinenone, phytoene	*Anabaena* sp., *Cylindrospermum* sp., *Microcystis* sp., *Nostoc* sp., *Oscillatoria* sp., *Phormidium* sp., *Synechococcus* sp., *Spirulina* sp., *Tolypothrix* sp.
Peptides	Peptides, proteins, free amino acids	*Aphanizomenon flos-aquae*, *Calothrix ghosei*, *Cylindrospermum muscicola*, *Hapalosiphon intricatus*, *Microcystis aeruginosa*, *Nostoc muscorum*, *Nostoc* sp.
Polysaccharides	β-Glucans, lipopolysaccharides, chitin, carrageenan	*A. platensis*, *Nostoc muscorum*, *Cylindrospermum muscicola*
Vitamins	Riboflavin, thiamine, ascorbic acid, nicotinic acid, cobalamine, phenothene, pyridoxine, folic acid	*Anabaena* sp., *Chroococcus mimulus*, *Nostoc* sp., *Microcystis pulverea*, *Oscillatoria jasorvensis*, *Arthrospira*, *Phormidium bijugatum*

Table 1.
Cyanobacterial strain metabolites [10].

doses. In addition, at highly controlled cultivation conditions, biomass with more stable chemical and functional characteristics can be obtained [3]. There are various types of molecules, among biostimulants, that can be extracted from cyanobacterial cells, and they include phytohormones, polysaccharides, protein hydrolysates, and amino acids [35]. Cyanobacterial strain metabolites are presented in **Table 1**.

3.1 Phytohormones

Auxin, cytokinin, gibberellic acid, ethylene, abscisic acid, salicylic acid, and jasmonic acid are examples of phytohormones known for their low molecular weight and signaling; their function is to coordinate many cellular activities in a plant cell [36]. The hormonal content of cyanobacteria and their capacity to stimulate endogenous hormone synthesis in treated plants have proven their ability to elevate plant growth. Obviously, like plant cells, some phytohormones are produced in these microorganisms [3].

3.1.1 Auxin

Auxin is a phytohormone that plays a key role in the precise control of plant growth and development; its effect on plants is well known. The main auxin in higher plants, indole acetic acid (IAA), has a structure consisting of an indole ring and an acetic acid side chain. IAA is basically a hetero-aromatic organic acid and exerts strong effects on plants; for example, it increases cell elongation, prevents or delays leaf abscission, and stimulates flowering and fruiting [36, 37]. Studies have shown that IAA produced in cyanobacterial species such as *Nostoc* spp., *Synechocystis* spp., and *Leptolyngbya* spp. improved the growth of wheat and rice; the highest concentration of the phytohormone has been observed during the colonization of plant roots. Furthermore, the role of auxins (IAA) and soluble AAs secreted by cyanobacteria in increasing soil microbial content and microbiome quality has also been proven [6].

3.1.2 Cytokinins

Cytokinins are one type of phytohormones, and their structure consists of N6-substituted adenine derivatives containing aromatic or isoprenoid side chains. They affect several plant physiological processes, such as morphogenesis, development of chloroplast, seed dormancy, leaf senescence, so they are very valuable in agriculture. Cytokinins cause cytoplasm division and are useful in reducing the adverse effects of abiotic stresses on plant growth [38, 39]. Similar to plants, the biosynthesis of cytokinins in cyanobacteria is carried out using isopentenyl transferases (IPTs); however, there are slight differences in the biosynthesis mechanism. It has been shown that the use of cyanobacterial supplements in the field has been led to the induction of adventitious roots and shoots on petiolar as well as internodal segments. According to the results of leaves, roots, and stems, explants of treated plants with cyanobacterial extract or cell suspension also showed successful regeneration [39, 40].

3.1.3 Gibberellic acid

Another phytohormone is gibberellic acid (GA3), which belongs to diterpenoid gibberellins. GA3 is a plant growth regulator; its function is to regulate plant growth and affect various developmental processes involving stem germination, elongation, flowering, and enzyme production. It has been reported that the extracellular extracts of *Scytonema hofmanni*, a cyanobacterium, contained gibberellin-like plant growth regulators, has reduced salt stress in rice seedlings [41, 42].

3.1.4 Abscisic acid

Abscisic acid (ABA) is another plant growth regulator; it is a natural sesquiterpene produced in plants and cyanobacteria. ABA inhibits growth and metabolism, improves fruit ripening and senescence, and also has remarkable effects on seed development and plant tolerance to biotic or abiotic stresses. The ability to produce this phytohormone in cyanobacteria such as *Nostoc muscorum*, *Trichormus variabilis,* and *Synechococcus leopoliensis* in culture media under salt stress has been demonstrated [43, 44].

3.1.5 Ethylene

This phytohormone is a gaseous hormone and its function is to regulate developmental processes like senescence, fruit ripening, cell division and elongation, and tolerance to biotic and abiotic stresses. Ethylene synthesis has been reported in cyanobacteria such as *Synechococcus* spp., *Anabaena* spp., *Nostoc* spp., *Calothrix* spp., *Scytonema* spp., and *Cylindrospermum* spp. [6, 45].

3.2 Polysaccharides

Cyanobacterial polysaccharides are promising plant biostimulants that can be found as cell envelope compounds, storage molecules, and extracellular polysaccharides (EPS). In general, cyanobacterial polysaccharides have three fates: to be combined with the cell wall, to be secreted as distinct structures (sheath, capsule, stalk), or to be released as mucilage [34, 46]. Maximum structural diversity and functional versatility are found in EPS; the functions of these polysaccharides, which interface with the surrounding environment, vary depending on the species, from a primary mechanism for survival in extreme environments to defense against toxins, heavy metals, predators, and other antagonists [47]. The key role of exopolysaccharides in soil aggregation is due to their gluing properties and binding to heavy metals and sodium ions, improving plant development in saline or contaminated soils [46].

Signaling pathways reliant on microbe-associated molecular patterns are common mechanisms through which the stimulatory properties of cyanobacterial polysaccharides may be explained. Soil enzymes such as β-glucanase and chitinase secreted by microorganisms can hydrolyze complex polysaccharides; then, receptors on plant membranes can recognize these neutral sugars from polysaccharides as microbial-derived compounds, providing organic carbon for the growth and development of beneficial microbes and also leading to form beneficent biofilms in the rhizosphere [6, 48]. Some ESP-producing cyanobacteria among different species of microalgae are *Spirulina platensis*, *Nostoc* spp., *Phormidium* spp., *Calothrix* spp., *Plectonema* spp. [6, 49].

3.3 C-phycocyanin

Cyano-phycocyanin (CPC) is one of the cyanobacterial bioactive pigments that are usually isolated from *Spirulina platensis* that has recently been identified with plant biostimulant properties [48, 50]. One function of CPC in the hydroponic growth medium is to adjust the microbial diversity and abundance; consequently, it stimulates actinobacteria and firmicutes. Therefore, the ability of CPC to stabilize plant growth-promoting bacteria and increase plant growth can represent its possible plant probiotic properties [6]. Since CPC is water-soluble, it can be a suitable compound to be considered as a biostimulant, but due to the sensitivity of CPC to high light, it must be used under controlled atmospheric growth conditions such as hydroponics and other vertical farming systems [6, 51].

3.4 Phenolic compounds and amino acids

One of the most principal classes of natural antioxidants are phenolic compounds, which are found in many organisms, including cyanobacteria. There are different amounts of polyphenolics such as caffeic, gallic, vanillic, ferulic acids, flavonoids, kaempferol, and quercetin in cyanobacterial extracts. The existence of polyphenols in these microorganisms demonstrated their ability to scavenge free radicals, chelate metals, and protect themselves against oxidative damage [42, 52]. Cyanobacterial strains that contain high amounts of polyphenols will achieve better ecological adaptation under different stress conditions by producing and releasing a wide range of bioactive compounds [42, 53]. Other organic compounds for applying as plant biostimulants to aid plant growth are amino acids that are found in cyanobacteria. Some of these microorganisms, such as *Arthrospira platensis*, showed high levels of L-amino acids, about 58% of their total protein content [54].

4. Role of cyanobacteria in plant health

Plants can benefit from cyanobacterial metabolites in various ways, such as enhancing their resistance to biotic and abiotic stressors and improving their growth and development. These metabolites are rich in bioactive substances and secondary metabolites that act as signal molecules to stimulate plant growth and stress tolerance [55, 56].

4.1 Cyanobacteria against plant abiotic stresses

Plant growth and development are adversely affected by abiotic stresses, which include extreme temperature, water scarcity or excess, high salt concentration, heavy metal toxicity, and ultraviolet exposure [57]. Plants spend most of their energy on maintenance, and vegetative and generative growth when the environment is favorable. But when they face harsh environmental conditions (such as cold, heat, drought, and salinity), they divert their resources to cope with stress, which reduces their growth and yield [58].

Cyanobacteria use different mechanisms to reduce abiotic stress in plants, which involve biochemical and molecular mechanisms such as increasing osmotic adjustment, proline accumulation, increased glutathione level, jasmonic acid and decreasing stress-related gene expression, and enhancing stress resistance gene synthesis and expression. Low-molecular-weight osmolytes, such as glycine betaine, amino acids, organic compounds, and various enzymes, also contribute to plant growth and development under stress conditions [59, 60].

Plants exposed to abiotic stresses show less damage when they interact with cyanobacteria. This occurs through both direct and indirect functions. The direct function is the effect of cyanobacteria on the soil quality, and the indirect function is the induction of specific responses in plants by cyanobacteria [57, 60]. Plants can cope with abiotic stresses better with the help of induced systemic tolerance (IST). This involves the production of phytohormones, such as IAA, cytokinins, and abscisic acid (ABA), which enable plants to withstand harsh environmental conditions. Additionally, the synthesis of antioxidants such as superoxide dismutase (SOD), peroxidase (POD), ascorbate peroxidase (APX), catalase (CAT), and glutathione reductase (GR) also reduces the damage caused by abiotic stresses [59, 61]. Another way to enhance plant resistance to abiotic stresses is to transfer genes from cyanobacteria that participate in fatty acid biosynthesis, carbon metabolism, and pigment biosynthesis [60].

4.2 Cyanobacteria against pests and pathogens (biocontrol)

Plant pests and pathogens are agents that cause disease and can be classified as bacteria, fungi, oomycetes, viruses, nematodes, or other pests. They are widely dispersed throughout the ecosystem and have the potential to negatively impact the fruit, stem, leaves, and root systems of several crops grown in all types of cultivation, leading to significant financial losses [62]. Some plants possess defense and resistance mechanisms, such as regulating gene expression, inducing or inhibiting particular metabolic pathways, and regulating signaling pathways to produce secondary metabolites with antibacterial and antioxidant properties. To reach the high desired production, however, the use of external protective agents is essential [58].

Numerous physiologically active and/or biocidal chemicals are known to be produced by cyanobacteria. These compounds may be able to counteract various pests and diseases or stimulate systemic and local resistance in plants. This presents a desirable and different strategy that does not have the drawbacks of chemical control, which is crucial for sustainable agriculture [60].

There is ample evidence that cyanobacteria have fungicidal properties. Numerous investigations, both *in vivo* and *in vitro*, have demonstrated the effectiveness of cyanobacteria against a variety of pathogenic fungi and oomycete, including species of *Fusarium* and *Aspergillus*. The primary method by which cyanobacteria lessen the detrimental effects of various pathogenic fungi on crops is by the production of chemicals known as antibiosis, which prevents the fungal growth and can even cause their death [60]. These metabolites exhibit a great deal of biological and chemical diversity. They may be classified as peptides, fatty acids, alkaloids, polyketides, macrolides, or another family of chemical compounds. Additionally, they can target various cell components. These chemicals have mostly been produced by filamentous cyanobacteria [63, 64].

Results regarding the use of cyanobacteria in the management of plant pathogenic nematodes are limited but extremely encouraging. When cyanobacteria come into touch with plant roots, they can trigger various defense mechanisms against nematodes. Similar to other pathogen families, antibiosis is the most extensively documented mechanism. It can cause nematodes to experience a variety of outcomes, including paralysis, death, accelerated egg hatching, and suppression of gall formation [60, 65].

Cyanobacteria can also be used to combat insects in agriculture. The generation of potent poisons is the primary means by which cyanobacteria fight insects. Some cyanobacteria species have the ability to trigger plant systemic resistance against insects in addition to producing poisons [60, 66].

5. Application and mode of action of cyanobacterial biostimulant

The method of application and the mechanisms by which cyanobacteria and their metabolites act as biostimulants are reviewed in this section.

5.1 Method of application

Biostimulants derived from cyanobacteria and microalgae have various forms of application, such as dry biomass, cell extracts, spent medium, or supernatant. The condition of the biostimulants determines the application method. They can be applied in different ways, such as soil drench or fertigation by irrigating the soil, seed treatments or primers for the plant seeds, and foliar spray for the leaf surface [67, 68]. Many factors influence the content and concentration of active compounds in cyanobacteria, such as species, application and extraction method, season, sampling site, culture and environmental conditions [69, 70]. The cyanobacterial bioactive metabolites may also deteriorate over long storage periods. Storage and shelf life are an

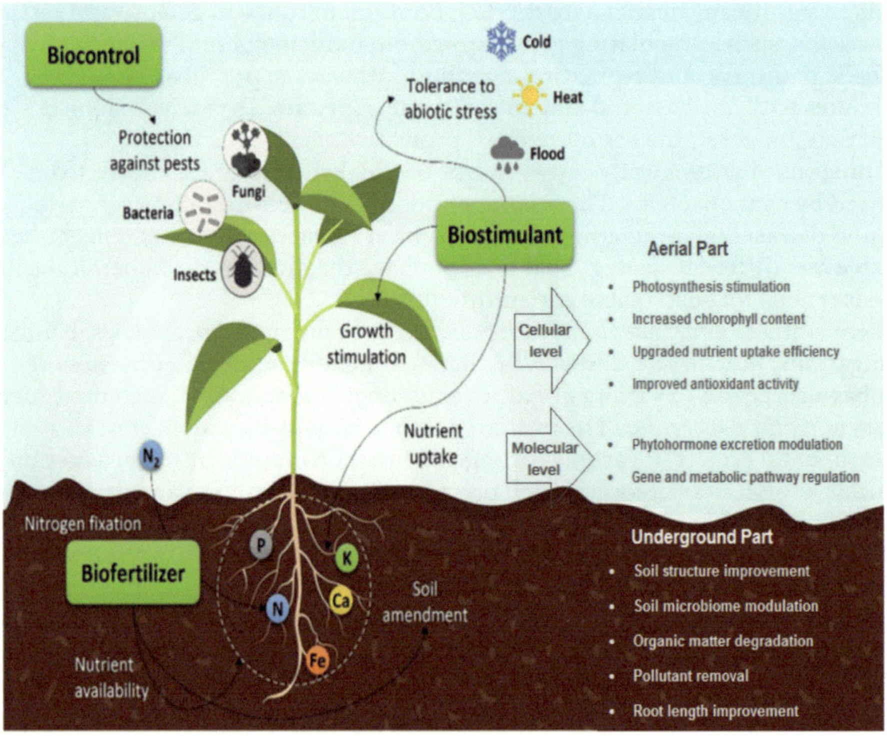

Figure 2.
Schematic of cyanobacterial bioproducts (biofertilizer, biostimulant, and biocontrol) and their impact on the crop and soil [60, 70].

important parameter that can affect root stimulation, and antioxidant and antibacterial activities of biostimulants were influenced by storage time, temperature, lighting conditions, and temperature [68, 71]. **Figure 2** shows the impact of cyanobacterial bioproducts on the crop and soil.

5.2 How cyanobacterial biostimulants act?

The effects of cyanobacterial biostimulants on plants are not well understood yet. Studying these mechanisms is complex and challenging. The variety and intricacy of compounds make it difficult to identify how biostimulants work. However, biostimulants are facilitators that can influence plants directly or indirectly. Direct effects include photosynthesis enhancement, nutrient uptake improvement, gene and metabolic pathway control, and phytohormone regulation, while indirect effects involve soil microbiome alteration, soil structure amelioration, and organic matter decomposition [72–75]. New methods such as omics approaches can help overcome the limitations in understanding how cyanobacterial biostimulants work [68].

6. Cyanobacteria: the effective key for space agriculture

To carry out space missions or settle in space, humans need some resources such as food, oxygen, which can be provided through space agriculture. Space agriculture means the cultivation and production of plants outside the earth [76]. Earth's environment is different from space and other bodies; plants that grow on the Earth and have adapted to its climate cannot grow outside the planet without any difficulties. The environment of space and other planets are generally extreme and the environmental parameters such as radiation exposure, magnetic field, light intensity, and microgravity exposure are in a different range from the Earth; therefore, it is very hard for plants to tolerate them [77, 78].

Using cyanobacteria is a novel and interesting method of growing plants in space. These photosynthetic microorganisms have survived in the extreme environments of the earth such as hot springs, deep seas, polar region [79] for billions of years, they have given life to the earth by photosynthesis, and they have the ability to deal with several stresses by producing secondary metabolites. Spatial stresses can increase the production of secondary metabolites by cyanobacteria and the use of cyanobacteria that grow up at this condition subsequently may enhance the growth and yield of plants [78]. Although some studies have been conducted on space agriculture and have investigated its efficiency, there are still several challenges that should be considered [80–82]. Investigating the challenges is necessary to state with certainty that using space agriculture in space settlements is a reliable approach.

7. Conclusion

Cyanobacteria are photosynthetic prokaryotes that can enhance plant performance, resilience, and sustainability. As biofertilizers, they can solubilize phosphate, improve soil quality and nutrient availability, and lower soil salinity. They can also enrich soil nitrogen by fixing atmospheric nitrogen, making them a useful supplement to biofertilizers. Moreover, cyanobacteria produce various bioactive compounds, such as phytohormones, polysaccharides, phenolic compounds, amino acids, and others, that can stimulate plant growth and development as biostimulants. By applying them through soil drenching or foliar spray, they can help plants cope with harsh environmental conditions, such as extreme temperatures, salinity, pests, and pathogens. Cyanobacterial metabolites may also indirectly benefit plants by inducing their defense system against biotic and abiotic stresses. Cyanobacteria can make bioactive molecules that boost plant growth and health even at low doses. They can also grow in controlled systems with stable composition and effects. These features make cyanobacteria a valuable bioresource for developing new and high-quality biostimulants for eco-friendly farming.

Acknowledgements

Thanks go to Ab-O-Aftab Zist Farayand (Water & Sun Bioprocess) R&D team.

Author details

Seyed Mojtaba Soleymani Robati
Faculty of Chemical Engineering, Department of Biotechnology, Tarbiat Modares University, Tehran, Iran

*Address all correspondence to: sm.soleymani@modares.ac.ir

References

[1] Paravar A, Piri R, Balouchi H, Ma Y. Microbial seed coating: An attractive tool for sustainable agriculture. Biotechnology Reports. 2023;**37**:e00781. DOI: 10.1016/j.btre.2023.e00781

[2] Nimsi KA, Manjusha K, Kathiresan K, Arya H. Plant growth-promoting yeasts (PGPY), the latest entrant for use in sustainable agriculture: A review. Journal of Applied Microbiology. 2023;**134**(2):lxac088. DOI: 10.1093/jambio/lxac088

[3] Múnera-Porras LM, García-Londoño S, Ríos-Osorio LA. Action mechanisms of plant growth promoting cyanobacteria in crops in situ: A systematic review of literature. International Journal of Agronomy. 2020;**2020**:1-9. DOI: 10.1155/2020/2690410

[4] Alvarez AL, Weyers SL, Goemann HM, Peyton BM, Gardner RD. Microalgae, soil and plants: A critical review of microalgae as renewable resources for agriculture. Algal Research. 2021;**54**:102200. DOI: 10.1016/j.algal.2021.102200

[5] Stal LJ. Nitrogen fixation in cyanobacteria. In: eLS. Chichester: John Wiley & Sons, Ltd.; 2015. pp. 1-9. DOI: 10.1002/9780470015902.a0021159

[6] Parmar P, Kumar R, Neha Y, Srivatsan V. Microalgae as next generation plant growth additives: Functions, applications, challenges and circular bioeconomy based solutions. Frontiers in Plant Science. 2023;**14**:1073546. DOI: 10.3389/fpls.2023.1073546

[7] Stewart WDP. Algal fixation of atmospheric nitrogen. Plant and Soil. 1970;**32**:555-588. DOI: 10.1007/BF01372896

[8] Kumar K, Mella-Herrera RA, Golden JW. Cyanobacterial heterocysts. Cold Spring Harbor Perspectives in Biology. 2010;**2**(4):a000315. DOI: 10.1101/cshperspect.a000315

[9] Bergman B, Gallon JR, Rai AN, Stal LJ. N_2 fixation by non-heterocystous cyanobacteria. FEMS Microbiology Reviews. 1997;**19**(3):139-185. DOI: 10.1016/S0168-6445(96) 00028-9

[10] Kollmen J, Strieth D. The beneficial effects of cyanobacterial co-culture on plant growth. Life. 2022;**12**(2):223. DOI: 10.3390/life12020223

[11] Zhang CC, Laurent S, Sakr S, Peng L, Bédu S. Heterocyst differentiation and pattern formation in cyanobacteria: A chorus of signals. Molecular Microbiology. 2006;**59**(2):367-375. DOI: 10.1111/j.1365-2958.2005.04979.x

[12] Krings M, Hass H, Kerp H, Taylor TN, Agerer R, Dotzler N. Endophytic cyanobacteria in a 400-million-yr-old land plant: A scenario for the origin of a symbiosis? Review of Palaeobotany and Palynology. 2009;**153**(1-2):62-69. DOI: 10.1016/j.revpalbo.2008.06.006

[13] Lee SM, Ryu CM. Algae as new kids in the beneficial plant microbiome. Frontiers in Plant Science. 2021;**12**:599742. DOI: 10.3389/fpls.2021.599742

[14] Adams DG, Duggan PS. Heterocyst and akinete differentiation in cyanobacteria. The New Phytologist. 1999;**144**(1):3-3. DOI: 10.1046/j.1469-8137.1999.00505.x

[15] Afkairin A, Ippolito JA, Stromberger M, Davis JG. Solubilization

of organic phosphorus sources by cyanobacteria and a commercially available bacterial consortium. Applied Soil Ecology. 2021;**162**:103900. DOI: 10.1016/j.apsoil.2021.103900

[16] Zhang M, Alva AK, Li YC, Calvert DV. Aluminum and iron fractions affecting phosphorus solubility and reactions in selected sandy soils. Soil Science. 2001;**166**(12):940-948. DOI: 10.1097/00010694-200112000-00008

[17] Chen YP, Rekha PD, Arun AB, Shen FT, Lai W-A, Young CC. Phosphate solubilizing bacteria from subtropical soil and their tricalcium phosphate solubilizing abilities. Applied Soil Ecology. 2006;**34**(1):33-41. DOI: 10.1016/j.apsoil.2005.12.002

[18] Prasanna R, Chaudhary V, Gupta V, Babu S, Kumar A, Singh R, et al. Cyanobacteria mediated plant growth promotion and bioprotection against fusarium wilt in tomato. European Journal of Plant Pathology. 2013;**136**:337-353. DOI: 10.1007/s10658-013-0167-x

[19] Prasanna R, Joshi M, Rana A, Shivay YS, Nain L. Influence of co-inoculation of bacteria-cyanobacteria on crop yield and C-N sequestration in soil under rice crop. World Journal of Microbiology and Biotechnology. 2012;**28**:1223-1235. DOI: 10.1007/s11274-011-0926-9

[20] Yandigeri MS, Meena KK, Srinivasan R, Pabbi S. Effect of mineral phosphate solubilization on biological nitrogen fixation by diazotrophic cyanobacteria. Indian Journal of Microbiology. 2011;**51**:48-53. DOI: 10.1007/s12088-011-0081-x

[21] Singh JS, Kumar A, Rai AN, Singh DP. Cyanobacteria: A precious bio-resource in agriculture, ecosystem, and environmental sustainability. Frontiers in Microbiology. 2016;7:529. DOI: 10.3389/fmicb.2016.00529

[22] Amini S, Ghadiri H, Chen C, Marschner P. Salt-affected soils, reclamation, carbon dynamics, and biochar: A review. Journal of Soils and Sediments. 2016;**16**:939-953. DOI: 10.1007/s11368-015-1293-1

[23] Nouri H, Chavoshi Borujeni S, Nirola R, Hassanli A, Beecham S, Alaghmand S, et al. Application of green remediation on soil salinity treatment: A review on halophytoremediation. Process Safety and Environmental Protection. 2017;**107**:94-107. DOI: 10.1016/j.psep.2017.01.021

[24] Meena MD, Narjary B, Sheoran P, Jat HS, Joshi PK, Chinchmalatpure AR, et al. Changes of phosphorus fractions in saline soil amended with municipal solid waste compost and mineral fertilizers in a mustard-pearl millet cropping system. Catena. 2018;**160**:32-40. DOI: 10.1016/j.catena.2017.09.002

[25] Deinlein U, Stephan AB, Horie T, Luo W, Xu G, Schroeder JI. Plant salt-tolerance mechanisms. Trends in Plant Science. 2014;**19**(6):371-379. DOI: 10.1016/j.tplants.2014.02.001

[26] Rath KM, Rousk J. Salt effects on the soil microbial decomposer community and their role in organic carbon cycling: A review. Soil Biology and Biochemistry. 2015;**81**:108-123. DOI: 10.1016/j.soilbio.2014.11.001

[27] Li H, Zhao Q, Huang H. Current states and challenges of salt-affected soil remediation by cyanobacteria. Science of the Total Environment. 2019;**669**:258-272. DOI: 10.1016/j.scitotenv.2019.03.104

[28] Rocha F, Lucas-Borja ME, Pereira P, Muñoz-Rojas M. Cyanobacteria as a

nature-based biotechnological tool for restoring salt-affected soils. Agronomy. 2020;**10**(9):1321. DOI: 10.3390/agronomy10091321

[29] Pade N, Hagemann M. Salt acclimation of cyanobacteria and their application in biotechnology. Life. 2014;**5**(1):25-49. DOI: 10.3390/life5010025

[30] Kirsch F, Klähn S, Hagemann M. Salt-regulated accumulation of the compatible solutes sucrose and glucosylglycerol in cyanobacteria and its biotechnological potential. Frontiers in Microbiology. 2019;**10**:2139. DOI: 10.3389/fmicb.2019.02139

[31] Rady MM, Taha SS, Kusvuran S. Integrative application of cyanobacteria and antioxidants improves common bean performance under saline conditions. Scientia Horticulturae. 2018;**233**:61-69. DOI: 10.1016/j.scienta.2018.01.047

[32] Singh S, Kant C, Yadav RK, Reddy YP, Abraham G. Cyanobacterial exopolysaccharides: Composition, biosynthesis, and biotechnological applications. In: Cyanobacteria. United State: Academic Press; 2019. pp. 347-358. DOI: 10.1016/B978-0-12-814667-5.00017-9

[33] Soltaniband V, Brégard A, Gaudreau L, Dorais M. Biostimulants promote plant development, crop productivity, and fruit quality of protected strawberries. Agronomy. 2022;**12**(7):1684. DOI: 10.3390/agronomy12071684

[34] Laroche C. Exopolysaccharides from microalgae and cyanobacteria: Diversity of strains, production strategies, and applications. Marine Drugs. 2022;**20**(5):336. DOI: 10.3390/md20050336

[35] Sánchez-Quintero Á, Fernandes SCM, Beigbeder J-B. Overview of microalgae and cyanobacteria-based biostimulants produced from wastewater and CO_2 streams towards sustainable agriculture: A review. Microbiological Research. 2023;**277**:127505. DOI: 10.1016/j.micres.2023.127505

[36] Mohamed ME, El Semary NA, Younis NS. Silver nanoparticle production by the cyanobacterium *Cyanothece* sp.: De novo manipulation of nano-biosynthesis by phytohormones. Life. 2022;**12**(2):139. DOI: 10.3390/life12020139

[37] Zhao Y. Auxin biosynthesis and its role in plant development. Annual Review of Plant Biology. 2010;**61**:49-64. DOI: 10.1146/annurev-arplant-042809-112308

[38] Kieber JJ, Schaller GE. Cytokinins. In: The Arabidopsis Book. United State: American Society of Plant Biologists; 2014. p. 12. DOI: 10.1199/tab.0168

[39] Uniyal S, Bhandari M, Singh P, Singh RK, Tiwari SP. Cytokinin biosynthesis in cyanobacteria: Insights for crop improvement. Frontiers in Genetics. 2022;**13**:933226. DOI: 10.3389/fgene.2022.933226

[40] Powell AE. The origin and early evolution of cytokinin signaling. Frontiers in Plant Science. 2023;**14**:1142748. DOI: 10.3389/fpls.2023.1142748

[41] Rodríguez A, Stella A, Storni M, Zulpa G, Zaccaro M. Effects of cyanobacterial extracellular products and gibberellic acid on salinity tolerance in *Oryza sativa* L. Saline Systems. 2006;**2**:1-4. DOI: 10.1186/1746-1448-2-7

[42] Kapoore RV, Wood EE, Llewellyn CA. Algae biostimulants: A critical look at microalgal biostimulants

for sustainable agricultural practices. Biotechnology Advances. 2021;**49**:107754. DOI: 10.1016/j.biotechadv.2021.107754

[43] Maršálek B, Zahradníčková H, Hronková M. Extracellular abscisic acid produced by cyanobacteria under salt stress. Journal of Plant Physiology. 1992;**139**(4):506-508. DOI: 10.1016/S0176-1617(11)80503-1

[44] Hartung W. The evolution of abscisic acid (ABA) and ABA function in lower plants, fungi and lichen. Functional Plant Biology. 2010;**37**(9):806-812. DOI: 10.1071/FP10058

[45] Allen CJ, Lacey RF, Binder Bickford AB, Beshears CP, Gilmartin CJ, Binder BM. Cyanobacteria respond to low levels of ethylene. Frontiers in Plant Science. 2019;**10**:950. DOI: 10.3389/fpls.2019.00950

[46] Santini G, Biondi N, Rodolfi L, Tredici MR. Plant biostimulants from cyanobacteria: An emerging strategy to improve yields and sustainability in agriculture. Plants. 2021;**10**(4):643. DOI: 10.3390/plants10040643

[47] Bhatnagar M, Bhatnagar A. Diversity of polysaccharides in cyanobacteria. In: Microbial Diversity in Ecosystem Sustainability and Biotechnological Applications. Singapore: Springer; 2019. pp. 447-496. DOI: 10.1007/978-981-13-83151_15

[48] Galinytė D, Balčiūnaitė-Murzienė G, Karosienė J, Morudov D, Naginienė R, Baranauskienė D, et al. Determination of heavy metal content: Arsenic, cadmium, mercury, and lead in cyano-phycocyanin isolated from the cyanobacterial biomass. Plants. 2023;**12**(17):3150. DOI: 10.3390/plants12173150

[49] Parwani L, Bhatt M, Singh J. Potential biotechnological applications of cyanobacterial exopolysaccharides. Brazilian Archives of Biology and Technology. 2021;**64**:e21200401. DOI: 10.1590/1678-4324-2021200401

[50] Varia J, Kamaleson C, Lerer L. Biostimulation with phycocyanin-rich Spirulina extract in hydroponic vertical farming. Scientia Horticulturae. 2022;**299**:111042. DOI: 10.1016/j.scienta.2022.111042

[51] Arahou F, Lijassi I, Wahby A, Rhazi L, Arahou M, Wahby I. Spirulina-based biostimulants for sustainable agriculture: Yield improvement and market trends. BioEnergy Research. 2023;**16**(3):1401-1416. DOI: 10.1007/s12155-022-10537-8

[52] Singh DP, Prabha R, Verma S, Meena KK, Yandigeri M. Antioxidant properties and polyphenolic content in terrestrial cyanobacteria. 3 Biotech. 2017;7:1-4. DOI: 10.1007/s13205-017-0786-6

[53] Yadav P, Singh RP, Rana S, Joshi D, Kumar D, Bhardwaj N, et al. Mechanisms of stress tolerance in cyanobacteria under extreme conditions. Stress. 2022;**2**(4):531-549. DOI: 10.3390/stresses2040036

[54] Mógor ÁF, de Oliveira Amatussi J, Mógor G, Bocchetti de Lara G. Bioactivity of cyanobacterial biomass related to amino acids induces growth and metabolic changes on seedlings and yield gains of organic red beet. American Journal of Plant Sciences. 2018;**9**(5):966-978. DOI: 10.4236/ajps.2018.95074

[55] Abo-Shady AM, Osman MEAH, Gaafar RM, Ismail GA, El-Nagar MMF. Cyanobacteria as a valuable natural resource for improved agriculture, environment, and plant protection. Water, Air, and Soil Pollution.

2023;**234**(5):313. DOI: 10.1007/s11270-023-06331-7

[56] Singh S. A review on possible elicitor molecules of cyanobacteria: Their role in improving plant growth and providing tolerance against biotic or abiotic stress. Journal of Applied Microbiology. 2014;**117**(5):1221-1244. DOI: 10.1111/jam.12612

[57] He M, He CQ, Ding NZ. Abiotic stresses: General defenses of land plants and chances for engineering multistress tolerance. Frontiers in Plant Science. 2018;**9**:1771. DOI: 10.3389/fpls.2018.01771

[58] Ferreira A, Bastos CRV, Marques-dos-Santos C, Acién-Fernandez FG, Gouveia L. Algaeculture for agriculture: From past to future. Frontiers in Agronomy. 2023;**5**:1064041. DOI: 10.3389/fagro.2023.1064041

[59] Munir N, Hanif M, Abideen Z, Sohail M, El-Keblawy A, Radicetti E, et al. Mechanisms and strategies of plant microbiome interactions to mitigate abiotic stresses. Agronomy. 2022;**12**(9):2069. DOI: 10.3390/agronomy12092069

[60] Poveda J. Cyanobacteria in plant health: Biological strategy against abiotic and biotic stresses. Crop Protection. 2021;**141**:105450. DOI: 10.1016/j.cropro.2020.105450

[61] Rajput VD, Harish, Singh RK, Verma KK, Sharma L, Quiroz-Figueroa FR, et al. Recent developments in enzymatic antioxidant defence mechanism in plants with special reference to abiotic stress. Biology. 2021;**10**(4):267. DOI: 10.3390/biology10040267

[62] Righini H, Francioso O, Quintana AM, Roberti R. Cyanobacteria: A natural source for controlling agricultural plant diseases caused by fungi and oomycetes and improving plant growth. Horticulturae. 2022;**8**(1):58. DOI: 10.3390/horticulturae8010058

[63] Righini H, Francioso O, Di Foggia M, Quintana AM, Roberti R. Preliminary study on the activity of phycobiliproteins against *Botrytis cinerea*. Marine Drugs. 2020;**18**(12):600. DOI: 10.3390/md18120600

[64] do Amaral SC, Xavier LP, Vasconcelos V, Santos AV. Cyanobacteria: A promising source of antifungal metabolites. Marine Drugs. 2023;**21**(6):359. DOI: 10.3390/md21060359

[65] Sithole N, Gupta S, Dube Z, Ogbe A, Van Staden J. Algae and cyanobacteria-based biostimulants in controlling plant-parasitic nematodes: A sustainable approach for crop protection. Phytoparasitica. 2023;**51**(4):803-813. DOI: 10.1007/s12600-023-01094-7

[66] Essack M, Alzubaidy HS, Bajic VB, Archer JAC. Chemical compounds toxic to invertebrates isolated from marine cyanobacteria of potential relevance to the agricultural industry. Toxins. 2014;**6**(11):3058-3076. DOI: 10.3390/toxins6113058

[67] Gitau MM, Farkas A, Balla B, Ördög V, Futó Z, Maróti G. Strain-specific biostimulant effects of chlorella and chlamydomonas green microalgae on medicago truncatula. Plants. 2021;**10**(6):1060. DOI: 10.3390/plants10061060

[68] Chabili A, Minaoui F, Hakkoum Z, Douma M, Meddich A, Loudiki M. A comprehensive review of microalgae and cyanobacteria-based biostimulants for agriculture uses. Plants. 2024;**13**(2):159. DOI: 10.3390/plants13020159

[69] Górka B, Korzeniowska K, Lipok J, Wieczorek PP. The biomass of algae and algal extracts in agricultural production. In: Algae Biomass: Characteristics and Applications. Switzerland: Springer; 2018. pp. 103-114. DOI: 10.1007/978-3-319-74703-3_9

[70] Márquez-Rocha FJ, Palma-Ramírez D, García-Alamilla P, López-Hernández JF, Santiago-Morales IS, Flores-Vela AI. Microalgae cultivation for secondary metabolite production. In: Microalgae—From Physiology to Application. United Kingdom: Intechopen; 2019. DOI: 10.5772/intechopen.88531

[71] Stirk WA, Bálint P, Vambe MM, Kulkarni MG, van Staden J, Ördög V. Effect of storage on plant biostimulant and bioactive properties of freeze-dried *Chlorella vulgaris* biomass. Journal of Applied Phycology. 2021;**33**(6):3797-3806. DOI: 10.1007/s10811-021-02596-9

[72] Ramakrishnan B, Maddela NR, Venkateswarlu K, Megharaj M. Potential of microalgae and cyanobacteria to improve soil health and agricultural productivity: A critical view. Environmental Science: Advances. 2023;**2**(4):586-611. DOI:10.1039/D2VA00158F

[73] Renuka N, Guldhe A, Prasanna R, Singh P, Bux F. Microalgae as multi-functional options in modern agriculture: Current trends, prospects and challenges. Biotechnology Advances. 2018;**36**(4):1255-1273. DOI: 10.1016/j.biotechadv.2018.04.004

[74] Kumar S, Korra T, Singh UB, Singh S, Bisen K. Microalgal based biostimulants as alleviator of biotic and abiotic stresses in crop plants. In: New and Future Developments in Microbial Biotechnology and Bioengineering. Netherland: Elsevier; 2022. pp. 195-216. DOI: 10.1016/B978-0-323-85577-8.00013-5

[75] Kumari M, Swarupa P, Kesari KK, Kumar A. Microbial inoculants as plant biostimulants: A review on risk status. Life. 2022;**13**(1):12. DOI: 10.3390/life13010012

[76] De Pascale S, Arena C, Aronne G, De Micco V, Pannico A, Paradiso R, et al. Biology and crop production in space environments: Challenges and opportunities. Life Sciences in Space Research. 2021;**29**:30-37. DOI: 10.1016/j.lssr.2021.02.005

[77] Zhang X, Li Z, Pang S, Jiang B, Yang Y, Duan Q, et al. The impact of cell structure, metabolism and group behavior for the survival of bacteria under stress conditions. Archives of Microbiology. 2021;**203**:431-441. DOI: 10.1007/s00203-020-02050-3

[78] Renaud C, Leys N, Wattiez R. Photosynthetic microorganisms, an overview of their biostimulant effects on plants and perspectives for space agriculture. Journal of Plant Interactions. 2023;**18**(1):2242697. DOI: 10.1080/17429145.2023.2242697

[79] Seckbach J, Chapman DJ, Garbary D, Oren A, Reisser W. Algae and cyanobacteria under environmental extremes: Final comments. Netherlands: Springer; 2007. DOI: 10.1007/978-1-4020-6112-7_42

[80] De Micco V, Aronne G, Caplin N, Carnero-Diaz E, Herranz R, Horemans N, et al. Perspectives for plant biology in space and analogue environments. npj Microgravity. 2023;**9**(1):67. DOI: 10.1038/s41526-023-00315-x

[81] Macário IPE, Veloso T, Frankenbach S, Serôdio J, Passos H, Sousa C, et al. Cyanobacteria as candidates to support Mars colonization: Growth and biofertilization

potential using Mars regolith as a resource. Frontiers in Microbiology. 2022;**13**:840098. DOI: 10.3389/fmicb.2022.840098

[82] Arai M. Cyanobacteria for space agriculture on Mars. Biological Sciences in Space. 2009;**23**(4):203-210. DOI: 10.2187/bss.23.203

Chapter 6

Cyanobacterial Toxins: Foes from the Water

Dijana Lalić

Abstract

This chapter is an introduction to the cyanobacterial (blue-green algae) ecology, with the main aim of better understanding the design of cyanobacterial blooms and cyanotoxins in the natural environments. Cyanobacteria are a diverse group of photoautotrophic organisms where their dominance represents a significant indicator of water quality. Several genera have the potential to produce toxins—hepatotoxins (microcystins, nodularins), cytotoxins (cylindrospermopsin), neurotoxins (saxitoxins, anatoxins, BMAA), dermatotoxins (lyngbyatoxin), and irritant toxins (lipopolysaccharide endotoxins). This chapter provides a concise and achievable summary of their negative impact on health and the environment, supplemented with tables and schemes that illustrate the ecology of cyanobacteria, the different types of cyanotoxins, and their health issues. The exposure routes are also discussed, which is particularly important due to the increasing eutrophication of water. It is emphasized that climate change, global warming, and increased eutrophication are responsible for cyanobacterial blooms. As a consequence, the risk they pose is likely to grow; accompanied by their ability to produce toxins, cyanobacteria represent an imminent danger to human and animal health. One of the primary goals of future research should be to share knowledge about cyanobacteria and cyanotoxins and to develop solutions for early detection and prevention of cyanobacterial bloom occurrence.

Keywords: cyanobacteria, cyanotoxins, toxicity, health, eutrophication, drinking water, recreational water

1. Introduction

Have you heard about cyanobacteria? How about blue-green algae? Both terms refer to prokaryotic organisms found in many water and terrestrial environments throughout the world. Cyanobacteria are especially abundant in shallow, warm, nutrient-rich, or polluted water low in oxygen, where under favorable environmental conditions their increased growth may form visible scums on water surfaces referred to as cyanobacterial blooms [1, 2], which is concerning in aquatic environments as the rapid increase of algae alters the quality of the water (**Figure 1**).

This group of prokaryotes has a remarkable ability to tolerate extreme environmental changes by producing a diverse range of secondary metabolites (e.g.,

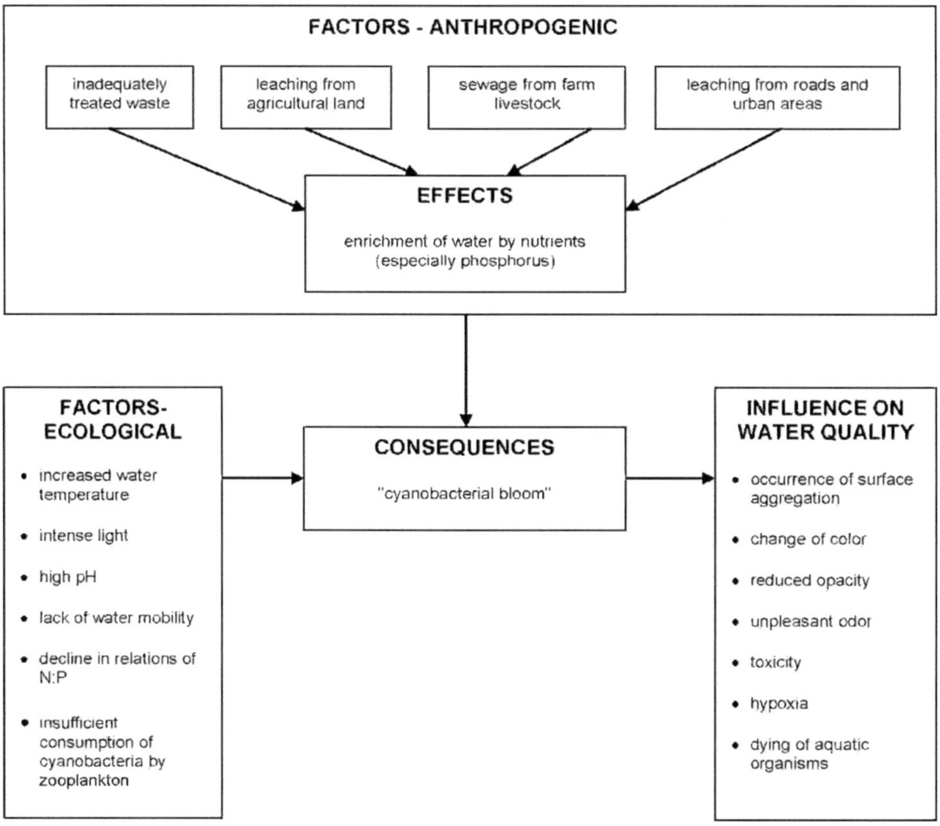

Figure 1.
Cyanobacterial blooms and their relation to the environment.

toxins—cyanotoxins and UV protective pigments—scytonemin and mycosporine-like amino acids), which gives them a competitive advantage [3]. We have all witnessed climate change and global warming over the past few decades (elevated temperature, increased atmospheric concentrations of carbon dioxide, elevated UV fluxes). The effects of global climate change and the associated accumulation of nutrients in water bodies by runoff from agricultural fertilizer, intensive farming practices, sewage discharge, and detergent usage are contributing to the accelerated decline in the quality of freshwater—eutrophication [1, 4]. Anthropogenic eutrophication of surface waters (**Figure 2**) implies rising nutrient levels (especially phosphorous but also nitrogen), low turbulence, stagnant water conditions, higher pH values, and higher temperature [4]. Drought can decrease water quality by concentrating pollutants (such as nutrients), and intense rain can wash fertilizers from crops, which are then discharged into water bodies. Resulting, cumulative conditions consequently stimulate the growth of cyanobacterial blooms in various geographic regions [5]. This accelerated growth of cyanobacteria in water bodies has severe impacts on ecosystem functioning—changes in biodiversity, light conditions or oxygen concentrations, and disturbances of relationships among organisms, which become a worldwide environmental problem. Approximately 50% of cyanobacterial secondary metabolites are known to produce extremely toxic metabolites known as cyanotoxins. Under these circumstances, cyanotoxins can reach high concentrations in waters and cause

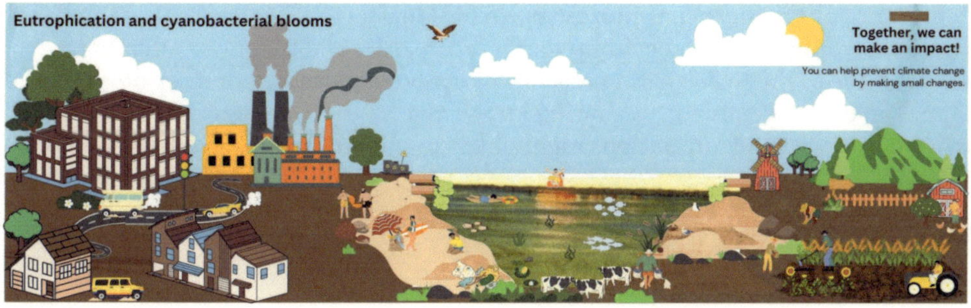
Eutrophication and cyanobacterial blooms
Together, we can make an impact!
You can help prevent climate change by making small changes.

Figure 2.
Eutrophication and cyanobacterial blooms (created by Author using Canva).

poisoning of animals and humans globally. Cyanotoxins can be intracellular, retained in cyanobacteria cells, and extracellular, released into the water during the life cycle and lysis [6]. Linked with negative environmental impacts large-scale cyanobacterial bloom events are classified as "harmful algal blooms" [7].

The current and expected future rise in cyanobacterial populations due to increasing anthropogenic eutrophication and global climate change [8, 9] suggests that further reports of poisoning events will occur. Mass occurrences of toxic cyanobacteria and their toxins in reservoirs represent a great challenge to produce safe drinking water and the development of advanced monitoring techniques [10]. The first step for cyanotoxin control is the prevention of the eutrophication process and reducing cyanobacterial blooms in water bodies. There is a necessity for improvements in the knowledge of cyanobacterial occurrence and ecology, and further, consequences of exposure to cyanotoxins. This chapter emphasizes emerging factors that contribute to the future expansion of cyanobacterial toxic blooms from aquatic ecosystems, and according to the newest data, from terrestrial environments, especially due to climate change, global warming, and anthropogenic eutrophication. Such information is crucial as the lack of knowledge about the toxic properties of cyanobacterial blooms has resulted in intoxication episodes worldwide, posing a problem that requires constant vigilance.

This comprehensive chapter presented the scenario of global warming and eutrophication, which will increase the risk of cyanobacterial bloom occurrence. Controlling the spread of cyanobacteria has become a significant global challenge. From a huge database of cyanobacterial occurrence and cyanotoxin poisonings [11], the number of research papers dealing with cyanotoxins seems to have increased exponentially over recent decades (from <2% before 1949 to over 72% after 2000). However, there are still unevenly distributed scientific researches and studies, with dominance in wealthier countries of the world. Also, despite improvements in analytical techniques, access to expensive equipment and standards, technical staff, and necessary handling skills will continue to limit cyanotoxin monitoring activity in wealthier countries. Without proper management, cyanobacteria can begin producing toxins. Cyanobacterial blooms that happened in the past and that are currently happening suggest that more research oriented toward cyanotoxin detection and purification system is needed. Standard procedures dealing with cyanotoxin detection should be standardized and implemented in the regulation system worldwide, and those procedures should be achievable for every country. Scientists should work on developing test kits for the detection of all types of cyanotoxins, not just for microcystin, as the most common cyanotoxin. Monitoring frequency (parameters such as chlorophyll-a, phycocyanin, temperature, pH, and turbidity) should be increased due to the widespread presence of cyanobacteria and their cyanotoxins [11]. There is an urgent requiring of sharing knowledge about cyanobacteria and their toxins to overcome the limitations highlighted in this study and encourage new behaviors.

2. Cyanotoxins

Cyanobacterial blooms with their production of potentially toxic secondary metabolites, cyanotoxins, present a worldwide threat to environmental and public health. Cyanotoxins are increasingly being viewed as contaminants of emerging concern (**Figure 3**). They are classified based on their target organs or cells. Cyanotoxins can affect the liver—hepatotoxins (microcystins, nodularin), nervous system—neurotoxins (anatoxin-a, homoanatoxin-a, anatoxin-a (S), saxitoxins and BMAA), cells—cytotoxins (cylindrospermopsin), or cause skin irritation—dermatotoxins (aplysiatoxin, debromoaplysiatoxin, lyngbyatoxin) and act like endotoxins (lipopolysaccharides) and other toxins [12, 13]. Cyanotoxins are recognized as one of the most lethal groups of biotoxins known [1], which could cause illness in humans

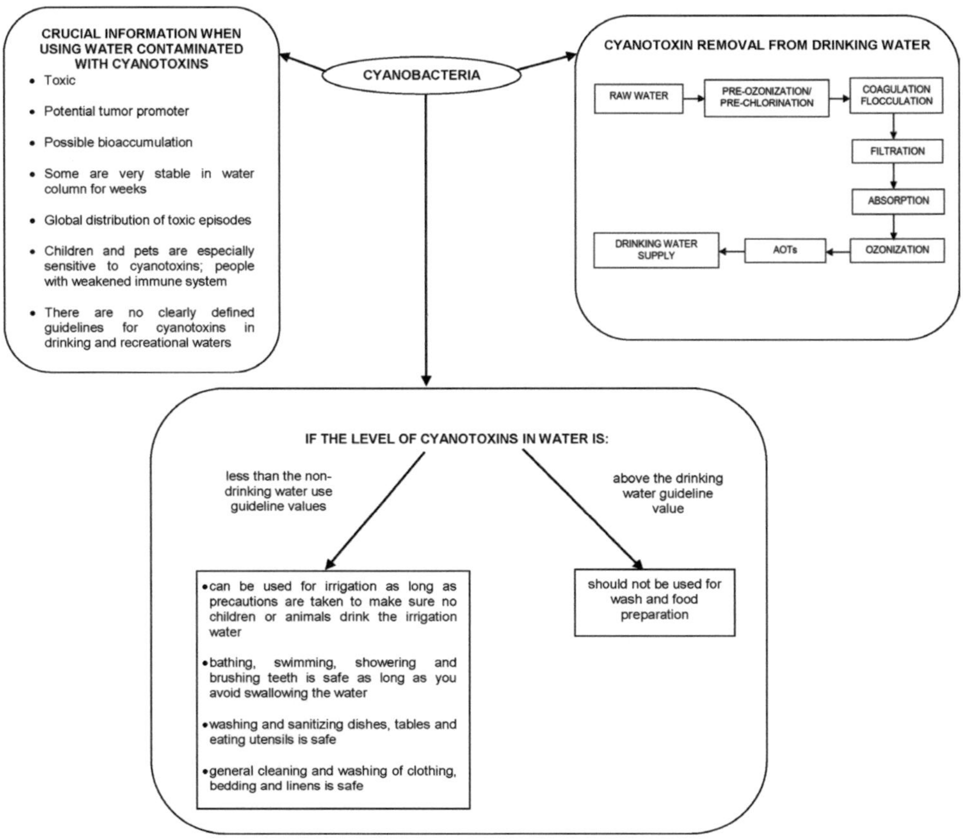

Figure 3.
Cyanobacteria and cyanotoxins in drinking/recreational water environments.

[14, 15], animals [16], and even death [17, 18]. Not all cyanobacterial blooms are toxic, and early surveys (determined by mouse intraperitoneal (*i.p.*) bioassay) indicated an incidence of 25–75% [6, 7]. The natural functions of their toxins remain to be fully understood; it may be an adaptation in resource-limiting environments as conferring competitive advantage and as cyanobacterial physiological aides [11].

Lately, many countries have been faced with cyanobacterial blooms affecting large areas with an increase in bloom incidence, followed by higher economic losses to aquaculture and tourism. Various cyanobacterial genera are known to produce toxins responsible for human and animal poisonings [11]. Microcystins, recognized as the most ubiquitous cyanotoxins [19], anatoxins, cylindrospermopsis, and other toxins, cause illness in humans and animals. The highest cyanotoxin levels are usually contained within the cells (intracellular toxins), in the cytoplasm, and toxin concentrations dissolved in the water (extracellular toxins) are rarely reported above a few μg/L [1]. The concentration of cyanotoxins significantly increases as a defense mechanism in stressful conditions (lack of nutrients/light) [20]. Dead cyanobacterial cells, whether at the end of their lifecycle or due to bloom control measures, can cause an increase in the concentration of extracellular toxins. Cyanotoxins are a concern when they are released into the water as they can be ingested by aquatic invertebrates, aquatic vertebrates [21–23], and even plants [24]. This can pose a potential health risk to humans and animals who consume contaminated food [25, 26]. Furthermore, children are particularly vulnerable to cyanobacterial toxins due to their lower body weight, behavior, and the toxic effects they can have on development [27].

When cyanobacterial cell concentrations are high due to bloom events, cyanotoxins can cause a noxious taste and odor in drinking and recreational water. They decay and resulting high biomass of cyanobacteria cause low oxygen events that kill fish, blocks sunlight preventing the growth of other algae and disrupting food webs [28]. During cyanobacterial blooming events, it is necessary to take caution of water-related activity (**Figure 3**). The presence of high levels of cyanotoxins in recreational and drinking water may cause a wide range of symptoms in humans (**Figure 4**), including fever, headaches, muscle and joint pain, blisters, severe oral and gastrointestinal inflammation, vomiting, mouth ulcers, and irritation of the skin and mucous membrane of the eyes, nose and throat, cyanosis, paralysis, and respiratory or cardiac arrest, potentially resulting in death. The health issues caused by cyanotoxins can occur within minutes to days after exposure in accordance with exposure route(s), the types and concentration of cyanotoxins, age and body weight, and health conditions of the affected person (e.g., associated diseases). In severe cases, seizures, cyanosis, paralysis, liver failure, respiratory arrest, and (rarely) death may occur [1, 11, 29]. Cyanobacteria can persist in water bodies for a long time, leading to prolonged exposure to subacute concentrations of cyanotoxins and the possibility of chronic health effects, including possible carcinogenic changes [30, 31], neurodegenerative diseases in humans [32], and harm to other living organisms, including invertebrates [33] and plants [34–36]. It can cause leaf necrosis, inhibition of photosynthesis and growth, and oxidative stress [34–36].

Based on the research [11], there were 183 recorded cyanotoxin poisonings of humans and animals reported worldwide, with most cases reported in North and Central America, followed by Europe and Australia/New Zealand. Microcystins were the most often recorded cyanotoxins worldwide (63%) followed by cylindrospermopsin (10%), anatoxins (9%), and saxitoxins (8%). Further, microcystins have been most commonly reported in cyanobacterial poisoning cases (42%),

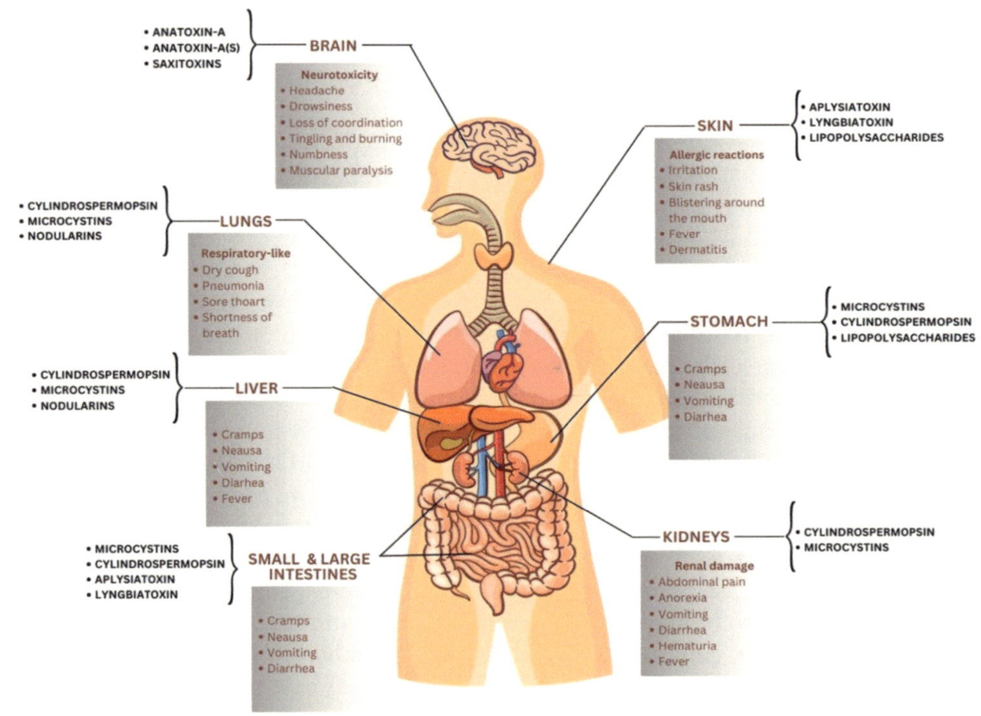

Figure 4.
Target organ of toxicity and health issues (created by Author using Canva).

and nodularin has been least often (2%). A total of 15% of all the poisoning cases were assigned due to unknown reasons and 17% due to not analyzing cyanotoxins. Poisoning events caused by cyanotoxins affected in 63% of cases only animals, whereas 32% of the investigated poisonings involved only humans. The presented data [11] suggest that future research should be orientated toward the creation of new, inexpensive, and more widely available analytical techniques for cyanotoxin detection.

2.1 Structure and characteristics of cyanotoxins

Cyanotoxins are very diverse regarding their chemical structure and toxicity (**Table 1** and **Figure 5**) [12, 37–40]. A structurally similar group of cyclic hepta- and pentapeptides is known as microcystins and nodularins, respectively [41, 42]. Microcystins (MCs) are the most ubiquitous toxins detected in cyanobacterial blooms and produced by various cyanobacterial genera *Aphanizomenon*, *Dolichospermum* (*Anabaena*), *Fischerella*, *Microcystis*, *Oscillatoria*, *Nostoc*, *Planktothrix*, *Synechococcus*, and *Trichodesmium* [19, 43, 44]. Microcystins act primarily through the inhibition of protein phosphatases 1 and 2A. The primary target cell for MCs is the liver [45]; however, these toxins can affect other tissues (kidney, reproductive tissue, colon, brain) [46]. Microcystin-LR (MC-LR) causes potent hepatotoxicity and it acts as a tumor promoter [47–50]. So far, about 250 variants of microcystin have been identified [51], but the most toxicological information is available for the MC-LR [52].

DOI: http://dx.doi.org/10.5772/intechopen.1005888

Toxins/structure (number of analogs)		Target organ and mechanism of action	Health effects	LD_{50} (*i.p.* mouse, µg/kg b.w.)	LD_{50} (oral, µg/kg b.w.)	Toxigenic genera	Reference
Hepatotoxins	Microcystins/cyclic heptapeptides (~250)	Irreversible inhibition of protein phosphatases (PP1 and PP2A), membrane integrity and conductance disruption; *primary site of action*: liver (also affect other tissues-kidney, reproductive tissue, colon, brain)	Nausea; vomiting; diarrhea; renal damage; hepatotoxic; tumor promoters; death (in some cases)/Immediate up to 24 hours	MC-LR-50; MC-LA-50; MC-YR-70; MC-RR-300-600; ([(6Z)-Adda] MC-RR)-1000	MC-LR-5000 (one strain of mice); 10,900 (another strain of mice); >5000 (in rats)	*Anabaenopsis, Aphanocapsa, Aphanizomenon, Arthrospira, Dolichospermum (Anabaena), Fischerella, Gloeotrichia, Hapalosiphon, Microcystis, Merismopedia, Nostoc, Oscillatoria, Phormidium, Planktothrix, Pleurocapsalean, Radiocystis Synechococcus, Snowella, Woronichinia*	[44, 46, 51, 53–58]
	Nodularins/cyclic pentapeptides (10)	Inhibition of protein phosphatases (PP1 and PP2A); *primary site of action*: liver	Hepatotoxic; tumor promoters; carcinogenic	30–60	ND	*Nodularia, Nostoc*	[30, 51, 59, 60]
Cytotoxins	Cylindrospermopsins/ guanidine alkaloids (3)	Irreversible inhibitor of protein biosynthesis; *primary site of action*: liver (also to kidneys, spleen, lungs, heart, intestine, thymus, skin)	Nausea; vomiting; bloody diarrhea; kidney damage; headache; dehydration; genotoxic/ Up to a week	200 (6 days)–2100 (24 h)	4400–6900 (2–6 days)	*Aphanizomenon, Chrysosporum, Cylindrospermopsis, Dolichospermum (Anabaena), Lyngbya, Oscillatoria, Raphidiopsis, Sphaerospermopsis, Umezakia*	[61–66]

Toxins/structure (number of analogs)		Target organ and mechanism of action	Health effects	LD_{50} (*i.p.* mouse, µg/kg b.w.)	LD_{50} (oral, µg/kg b.w.)	Toxigenic genera	Reference
Neurotoxins	Anatoxin-a/alkaloids (8)	Postsynaptic, depolarizing neuromuscular blockers, binds irreversibly to the nicotinic acetylcholine receptors; *primary site of action*: nerve synapse	Tingling in fingers and toes; dizziness; convulsions; paralysis; muscle fasciculation; gasping; death (in some cases)/ Immediate up to 1 to 2 h	200–375	>5000	*Aphanizomenon, Arthrospira, Cylindrospermum, Dolichospermum (Anabaena), Microcystis, Oscillatoria, Planktothrix, Raphidiopsis, Tychonema*	[30, 38, 53, 56, 57, 59, 60, 67–71]
	Homoanatoxin-a/ alkaloids (1)	Similar to anatoxin-a, cause a potent neuromuscular blockade; *primary site of action*: nerve synapse	Staggering; gasping; muscle fasciculation; convulsions; coma; cyanosis; hyper salivation; death	250–330	ND	*Phormidium (Oscillatoria), Raphidiopsis*	[30, 72–74]
	Anatoxin-a(S)/guanidine methyl phosphate ester (1)	Irreversibly inhibits acetylcholinesterase, nerve hyper-excitability; *Primary site of action*: peripheral nervous system	Hyper salivation; diarrhea; paralysis; asphyxiation; decreased movement; exaggerated abdominal breathing; cyanosis; convul-sion; and ultimately death/ Survival time of 10–30 min	20–40	ND	*Dolichospermum (Anabaena)*	[70, 75–79]
	Saxitoxins/carbamate alkaloids (56)	Binds and blocks the sodium channels inhibiting nerve axon conduction; *primary site of action*: nerve axons	Numbness around mouth; spreading to arms and hands; respiratory muscle paralysis; difficulty breathing; death/ Immediate up to 24 h	5–30	263	*Aphanizomenon, Lyngbya, Dolichospermum, Planktothrix, Phormidium, Scytonema, Geitlerinema, Raphidiopsis, Cuspidothrix, Cylindrospermopsis*	[37, 80–85]
	b N-methylamino-L-alanine (BMAA)/amino acids (1)	*Alkaloid precursors; primary site of action*: motor neurons	Neurodegenerative agents	ND	ND	*Aphanizomemon, Cylindrospermopsis, Dolichospermum, Microcystis, Nodularia, Planktothrix (Oscillatoria), Synechococcus, Synechocystis*	[60, 86]

DOI: http://dx.doi.org/10.5772/intechopen.1005888

Toxins/structure (number of analogs)		Target organ and mechanism of action	Health effects	LD_{50} (*i.p.* mouse, µg/kg b.w.)	LD_{50} (oral, µg/kg b.w.)	Toxigenic genera	Reference
Dermatotoxins (irritants)	Lyngbyatoxin/modified cyclic dipeptide (3)	Protein kinase C activators; *primary site of action*: skin, gastro-intestinal tract	Inflammatory agent; dermatitis; necrosis; blisters; dermatoxins; tumor promoters	250 µg/kg (LD_{100})	ND	*Lyngbya, Schizotrix, Oscillatoria*	[29, 60, 87, 88]
	Aplysiatoxin/phenolic bislactones (>2)	Protein kinase C activators; *primary site of action*: skin	Inflammatory agent; dermatitis; necrosis; blisters; dermatoxins; tumor promoters	300	ND	*Lyngbya, Schizotrix, Oscillatoria*	[29, 87, 88]
	Debromoaplysiatoxin/ phenolic bislactones	Inflammatory toxins operate through mechanisms similar to those of phorbol esters *primary site of action*: skin	Inflammatory agent; dermatitis; blisters and necrosis in mammals	107–117 µg/kg	ND	*Lyngbya, Schizotrix, Oscillatoria*	[60, 89]
Endotoxins (irritants)	Lipopolysaccharides/ lipopolysaccharides (3)	LPS form complexes with proteins and phospholipids; *primary site of action*: affects any exposed tissue (skin and mucosa)	Inflammatory agents; headache; fever; skin irritations; gastrointestinal, allergic and respiratory reactions	40,000–190,000	ND	All cyanobacteria	[1, 90]

Abbreviations: i.p. = intraperitoneal exposure; LD50-lethal dose, which causes the death of 50% of tested animals (µg/kg body weight); ND = not determined.

Table 1.
Main toxicological data of cyanotoxins.

Nodularins (NODs) are highly toxic pentapeptides with a similar mechanism of toxicity to MCs (**Table 1**) [91, 92]. NODs are predominantly produced by *Nodularia spumigena* [93, 94]. Nodularin expresses toxicity through the inhibition of serine-threonine phosphatases, thus impairing signal transduction [49]. These potent toxins are able to cause oxidative stress in cells, which may promote hepatotoxicity and carcinogenicity [95]. Their production is generally limited to saline/brackish

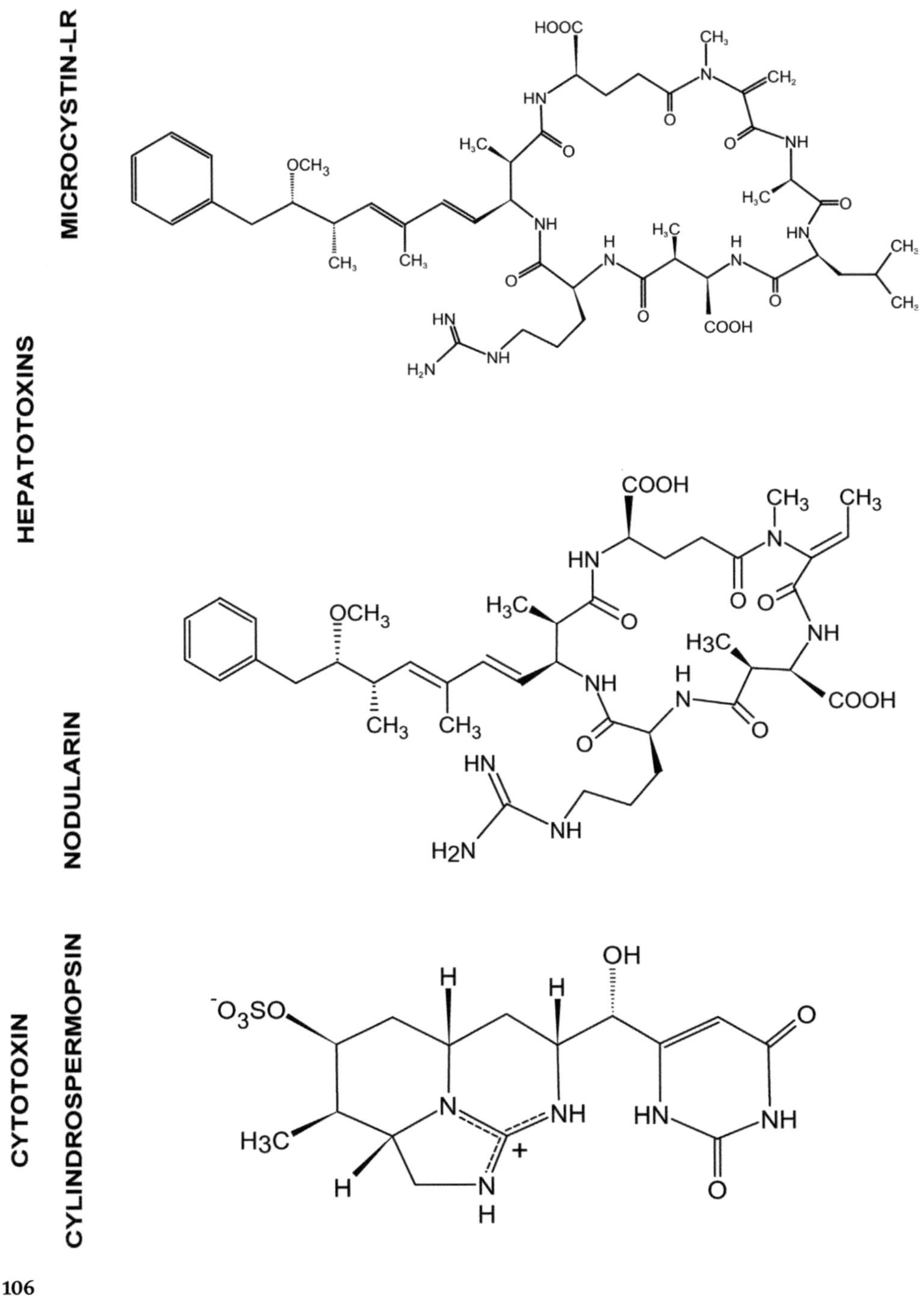

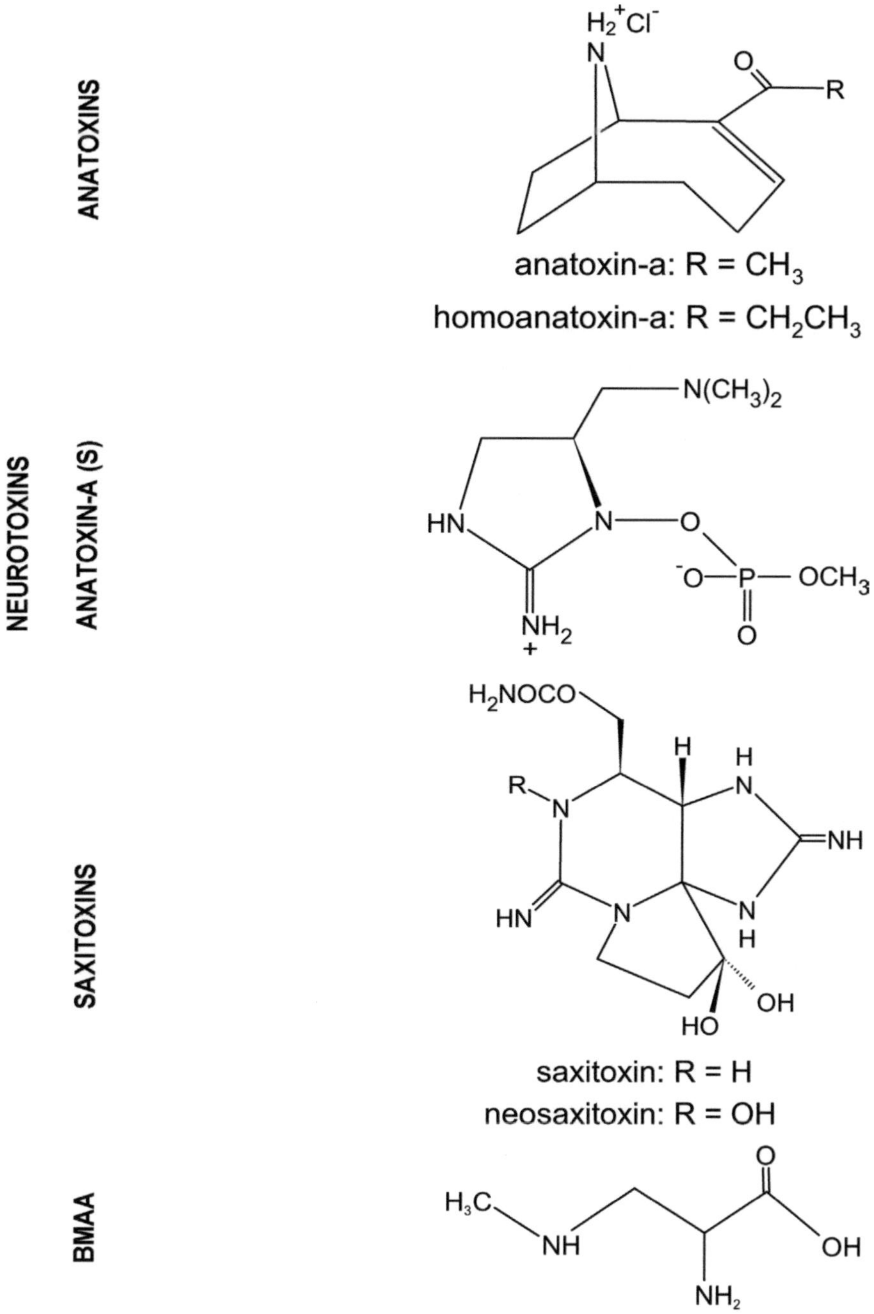

Figure 5.
Molecular structures of cyanobacterial toxins (created by Author using ChemSketch).

environments and terrestrial symbiotic associations [96]. More data from the cumulative or synergistic effects of NODs are urgently needed.

Cylindrospermopsin (CYN) is a highly toxic guanidine alkaloid that may act through disruption of the synthesis of glutathione and protein and cytochrome P450. This toxic compound is known to cause a range of harmful effects in mammals, including hepatotoxicity, neurotoxicity, genotoxicity, cytotoxicity, and carcinogenicity [97, 98]. Cylindrospermopsin was chemically characterized from the species *Raphidiopsis raciborskii* (formerly *Cylindrospermopsis raciborskii*) [61, 64], and two congeners, 7-epi-cylindrospermopsin and deoxycylindrospermopsin, have been identified [62, 99]. Besides genera *Raphidiopsis* (also known as *Cylindrospermopsis*) [62], a number of cyanobacterial genera (**Table 1**) e.g., *Umezakia* [100], *Aphanizomenon* [101], *Lyngbya* [66], *Anabaena* [65], *Chrysosporum* [63], *Dolichospermum* (*Anabaena*), *Oscillatoria*, *Phormidium*, and *Planktothrix* [98] have been found to produce CYN. These cyanobacterial species occur mostly in tropical or subtropical regions [99, 102, 103], usually concentrated several meters below the water surface increasing the risk in drinking water supplies since water is usually drawn into treatment plants from that depth [68].

Saxitoxins (STX) are a group of tricyclic neurotoxic alkaloids [104] that have gained notoriety as paralytic shellfish poisons. These toxins are known to accumulate in shellfish *Saxidomus giganteus*, from which the first identification of saxitoxins was made [104]. STX is considered among the most toxic compounds of biological origin described to date [84], with an LD50 of 5 μ kg^{-1} in mice (*i.p.*) [37]. They cause symptoms like respiratory muscle paralysis. In freshwaters, STXs are mainly produced by filamentous cyanobacterial species belonging to the orders *Nostocales* (*Dolichospermum circinale* (formerly *Anabaena circinalis*), *Aphanizomenon gracile*, *Cuspidothrix issatschenkoi*, *Raphidiopsis raciborskii*, *Raphidiopsis brookii*, *Scytonema* sp.), and *Oscillatoriales* (*Lyngbya wollei*, *Geitlerinema* spp., *Phormidium uncinatum*) [82, 84, 105, 106]. STX analogs have been identified from the freshwater mat-forming cyanobacteria *Lyngbya wollei* [107–109]. Neosaxitoxin (NSTX) is a variant of saxitoxin with an additional hydroxyl group at the N1 position of the 1,2,3 guanidinium (N1-OH). Both toxin variants block the inward flow of sodium ions across the membrane channels [110].

Anatoxin-a (ATX-a) is a type of secondary bicyclic amine alkaloid [70] that is produced by several different genera of cyanobacteria—*Dolichospermum* (*Anabaena*) [67, 111], *Anabaena* [59, 112, 113], *Aphanizomenon* [59, 114, 115], *Oscillatoria* [59, 116, 117], *Planktothrix* [118], *Cylindrospermum* [59, 79], *Microcystis* [119], *Raphidiopsis* [74], *Nostoc* [120], *Phormidium* [121], *Arthrospira* [122], *Hydrocoleum* [123], and *Cuspidothrix* [124–126]. ATX-a is a potent postsynaptic depolarizing neuromuscular blocking agent and causes neurotoxic effects in vertebrates, including muscle fasciculation, gasping, decreased movement, abdominal breathing, cyanosis, convulsions, and death within minutes to hours by respiratory arrest [37, 79]. ATX-a degrades rapidly, with a half-life of 1–2 hours [38]. A methylene analog with a propyl group replacing the acetyl group, homoanatoxin-a, was isolated from *Phormidium* (*Oscillatoria*) *formosa*. Homoanatoxin-a mimics acetylcholine and binds to the nicotinic-acetylcholine receptors with higher affinity than acetylcholine [67].

Anatoxin-a(S) (ATX-a(S)) is a unique phosphate ester of a cyclic Nhydroxyguanine, which is produced only in species of *Dolichospermum* genus (*D. lammermannii*, *D. flos-aquae*, *D. spiroides*) [75, 76, 79, 108]. Anatoxin-a(S) is different in structure and toxicity mechanism from ATX-a [39] and was named due to salivation by intoxicated animals [64]. The clinical signs of toxicosis are similar to anatoxin-a, characterized by excessive salivation, watery eyes, nasal discharge, tremors, loss of balance, cyanosis, convulsion, muscle twitching and cramping, diarrhea, and seizures leading to death [75, 105, 110, 127]. ATX -a(S) toxicosis has been reported in dogs, pigs, and geese, with survival times ranging from 5 to 30 minutes. So far, there have not been detected structural variants. It is rare detection can be due to chemical instability [76].

In Ref. [128], for the first time, lipopolysaccharides (LPS) from the cyanobacterial species *Anacystis nidulans* were isolated. Lipopolysaccharides form a crucial component of the cell wall in Gram-negative bacteria, which includes cyanobacteria [129]. These complex molecules play a vital role in regulating the immune response. Lipopolysaccharides are pyrogenic, dermatoxic compounds that cause allergenic reactions in humans and animals [130]. This is also a tumor promoter due to the potent activation of protein kinase C. The largest producer of these toxins is *Lyngbya sp*. (*Lyngbya majuscula* and *L. wollei*), which also produce a large array of these toxins [131]. Three congeners of lyngbyatoxin have been isolated—lyngbyatoxin A, B, and C [132]. Aplysiatoxin and analogs thereof have been isolated from *Lyngbya majuscula* [133], *Schizothrix calcicola* [89], *Oscillatoria nigro-viridis* [89], and *Trichodesmium erythraeum* [134]. Naturally occurring aplysiatoxin analogs have also been identified [89, 134]. Similar to lyngbyatoxin, aplysiatoxins induce contact dermatitis through the activation of protein kinase C. Cyanobacterial LPS has a smaller toxic effect than LPS of other bacteria [135].

Beta-N-methylamino-L-alanine (BMAA) is a non-proteinogenic amino acid produced by diverse aquatic and terrestrial cyanobacteria [136]. BMAA has been shown to be neurotoxic in a variety of animal models [32]. Also, there is a possible connection with the induction of several neurodegenerative diseases, including amyotrophic lateral sclerosis, Parkinsons' disease, and dementia [32]. The only study about known exposure of humans to BMAA involves a terrestrial food web [137]. A recent case study [138] detected BMAA in postmortem olfactory tissues of individuals with varying stages of Alzheimer's disease.

3. Exposure routes of cyanotoxins

Aquatic cyanobacterial strains produce a wide array of potent cyanotoxins able to cause environmental problems and health issues. Exposure routes to toxic cyanobacterial blooms (**Figure 6**) are mostly introduced through ingestion of contaminated drinking water [30, 139, 140], contaminated fish or shellfish [141, 142] and food and dietary supplements [143], recreational use of lakes and rivers [144], inhalation of aerosols [145, 146], receiving dialysis with contaminated water (e.g., which was documented in Brazil) [147, 148], or irrigation of agricultural products with contaminated water [35, 147, 149, 150]. Potential consequences of cyanotoxin exposure range from mere nuisances to serious health threats in humans and animals, even with fatal outcomes [11, 17, 18].

Incidents of human and animal intoxications, after exposure to toxic blooms through drinking and recreational waters, have been documented worldwide [11]. Animals have been affected mostly through ingestion and direct exposure to cyanotoxins in Australia, Switzerland, Sweden, Scotland, the USA, Kenya, South Africa, and Russia [11]. From the extensive database, which is provided by Svirčev et al. [11], Australia has experienced the highest incidence and severity of cyanotoxin poisonings where the Darling River experienced a massive proliferation of *D. circinalis* (formerly *Anabaena circinalis*), which led to the death of 10,000 livestock [151]. Death cases of humans have been documented through hemodialysis reported in Portugal [152, 153], USA [154], as well as in Australia, where 149 people were hospitalized after ingestion of water from reservoir tank contaminated with cyanobacterial bloom (formerly) *C.*

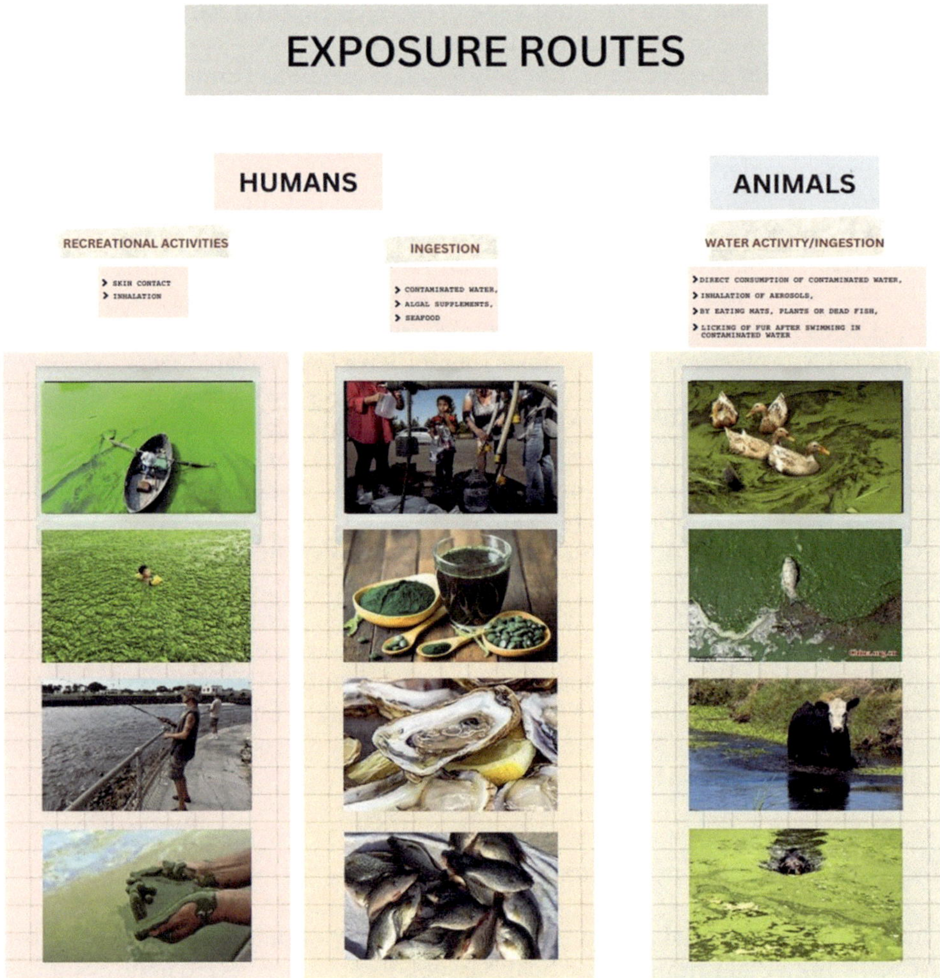

Figure 6.
Exposure routes of cyanotoxins (created by Author using Canva). Source for the photographs used in schematic presentation of this figure (from left to right): https://www.chinausfocus.com/energy-environment/chinese-scientists-make-landmark-discovery-in-fight-against-toxic-algae-blooms; https://www.theoxygenproject.com/habs/; https://www.tcpalm.com/story/news/local/indian-river-lagoon/health/2018/08/20/algae-affect-people-who-eat-local-fish/1023490002/; https://www.theoxygenproject.com/habs/; https://newrepublic.com/article/154799/frightening-spread-toxic-algae; https://www.fda.gov/files/BlueGreenAlgaeSpirulinaMicrocystins1600x900_0.png; https://world.dan.org/wp-content/uploads/2020/07/paralytic-shellfish-poisoning-PSP-oysters-178781671-DAN-256x229-1.jpg; https://www.tcpalm.com/story/news/2018/07/18/floridas-polluted-waters-algae-eating-fish-linked-als-and-alzheimers/791158002/; https://www.nbcnews.com/id/wbna24467924; http://www.china.org.cn/photos/2015-07/13/content_36047492_3.htm; https://www.cdc.gov/habs/illness-symptoms-freshwater.html; https://www.housebeautiful.com/lifestyle/kids-pets/a28723484/blue-green-algae-killing-dogs/.

raciborskii [155]. Furthermore, 2000 persons, of which 88 died, manifested gastrointestinal symptoms after drinking water from the newly built dam reservoir in Brazil contaminated with cyanobacterial toxins [155, 156]. In addition, cases of cyanobacterial intoxication through the food chain have been documented in the literature. Cyanotoxin presence in water used for irrigation may have considerable impact on the growth and development of plants [34, 35], and through the food chain, it can potentially affect human health [11, 157]. The toxic effects of BMAA have mainly been reported through ingestion. According to the most recent study [149], BMAA has been found in the irrigation water and grains of certain cereal plants from farmlands that are irrigated with Nile River water (Egypt). BMAA was also accumulated in most vegetable plants in the concentrations correlated with BMAA concentrations detected in relevant irrigation water sites [149, 150]. The highest levels were obtained in zucchini fruits, followed by watercress, tomato fruits, green pepper fruits, radish leaves, and pea fruits [149]. It has been found that long-term intake of BMAA through diet is linked to the development of neurodegenerative disorders in humans [158]. However, recent studies suggest that exposure to BMAA through inhalation may also provide risks for neurodegenerative issues [137]. Furthermore, cyanotoxins can be accumulated in the fishes and mussels exposed to cyanobacterial blooms. Annually, around 2000 cases of human poisoning are reported globally, with a 15% mortality rate caused by the consumption of fish or shellfish that have fed on marine dinoflagellates, which are producers of saxitoxins [159]. Hepatotoxicosis and neurotoxicosis are the most common syndromes caused by toxic cyanobacterial blooms. After acute contact with cyanobacterial bloom, possible health problems are weakness, diarrhea, vomiting, abdominal pain, skin irritation, irritation in the eyes, nose, and throat, asthmatic attacks, muscle tremors, nausea, tingling in fingertips and toes, dizziness, blurred vision, headache, fever, hypoxia, cyanosis, paralysis, and respiratory or cardiac arrest resulting in death [1]. Chronic exposure to low cyanotoxin concentration leads to liver damage [155] and the development of primary liver cancer, which is proven in China [15, 160], and colorectal cancer in the town of Haining [161], and recently, in a small clinical study, where MC/NOD and CYN were detected in all patients with hepatocellular carcinoma [162].

4. How to prevent the cyanobacterial blooms in water bodies and how to protect yourself and your companion animals

Preventing the appearance of cyanobacterial blooms is the most effective method for avoiding contamination of water with cyanotoxins. To help reduce cyanobacterial blooms from forming, it is important to:

- reduce the amount of nutrients flowing into nearby water bodies by using only the recommended amounts of fertilizers on the farm, yard, and garden;
- prevent wastewater from leaking into nearby water bodies by ensuring proper maintenance of the septic system;
- reduce discharges from municipal and industrial wastewater treatment plants through biological, physical, or chemical measures.

Considering all that has been stated before, some precautionary steps need to be taken to prevent illness in your family and companion animals.

If you see signs of a bloom (e.g., smells bad—earthy odors, such as rotting plants; looks discolored; has foam, scum on the surface; has dead fish/other animals on its shore, etc), stay out of the water. Avoid eating fish and shellfish from water suspected of being contaminated with cyanobacteria. People should consult with a healthcare provider before taking food supplements containing cyanobacteria or giving them to a child. Do not fish, swim, boat, or play water sports in that area. Also, protect your pets and livestock from getting sick by keeping them away from water with possible cyanobacteria. Do not let animals drink the water, get into the water, lick or eat mats (of cyanobacteria), or eat dead fish, shells, and shrimps on the shore.

Nonetheless, if you or your companion animals do go in water possibly contaminated with cyanobacterial bloom, rinse yourself and your pets immediately afterward with tap water. Do not let pets lick their fur until they have been rinsed.

5. Conclusion

Cyanobacteria are charging ahead forcefully, supported by climate change, global warming, increased industrialization, and urban and farm pollution—eutrophication. This continues to affect human health as well as causing wildlife and domestic animal deaths through ingestion, inhalation, or dermal pathways. The infrequent research on cyanotoxins (aside from MCs) despite the high risks of human and animal intoxication cases, highlights the growing need for the development and application of effective water monitoring and management strategies. This is crucial for preventing cyanobacterial bloom occurrence and should be affordable for all geographic regions. In future research, it is important to share knowledge of this potential risk and how to take appropriate precautions to safeguard human health and companion animals and the health of the environment. Further, developing robust, precise, and inexpensive analytic techniques for the early detection of cyanotoxins should be one of the main aims of modern research. Given unequally distributed investigations and scientists, but equally distributed cyanotoxins in water bodies worldwide, we recommend introducing projects and workshops that would connect different countries and provide knowledge to both, the scientific community and those with a lower level of education. Because—Every little step is a huge step forward.

Acknowledgements

This work was supported by the Ministry of Science, Technological Development and Innovation of the Republic of Serbia (Grants No. 451-03-66/2024-2103/200125 & 451-03-65/2024-2103/200125).

I would like to express my deepest appreciation to my dear colleague Dr. Gorenka Bojadžija Savić for helpful contributions, constructive advice, and insightful suggestions.

Conflict of interest

The author declares no conflict of interest.

Abbreviations

ATX-a	anatoxin-a
ATX-a(S)	anatoxin-a(S)
BMAA	β-N-methylamino-L-alanine
CYN	cylindrospermopsin

MC	microcystin
MC-LR	microcystin-LR
NOD	nodularin
NSTX	neosaxitoxin
STX	saxitoxin
LPS	lipopolysaccharides

Author details

Dijana Lalić
Faculty of Sciences, Department of Biology and Ecology, University of Novi Sad, Novi Sad, Serbia

*Address all correspondence to: dijana.pantelic@dbe.uns.ac.rs

References

[1] Chorus I, Bartram J, editors. Toxic Cyanobacteria in Water: A Guide for their Public Health Consequences, Monitoring and Management. London, New York: Published on behalf of WHO by E&FN Spon; 1999

[2] Oberholster PJ, Botha A-M, Grobbelaar JU. *Microcystis aeruginosa*: Source of toxic microcystins in drinking water. African Journal Biotechnology. 2004;**3**:159-168

[3] Lalić D, Meriluoto J, Zorić M, Dulić T, Mirosavljević M, Župunski M, et al. Potential of cyanobacterial secondary metabolites as biomarkers for paleoclimate reconstruction. Catena. 2020;**185**:104283

[4] Reynolds CS. Cyanobacterial water blooms. In: Callow JA, editor. Advances in Botanical Research. London: Academic Press; 1987. pp. 67-143

[5] Sivonen K, Niemala SI, Niemi RM, Lepisto L, Luoma TH, Rasanen LA. Toxic cyanobacteria (blue green algae) in Finnish fresh and coastal waters. Hydrobiologia. 1990;**190**:267-275

[6] Codd GA. The Toxicity of Benthic Blue-Green Algae in Scottish Freshwaters. Marlow, UK: Foundation for Water Research; 1995

[7] Chorus I. Introduction: Cyanotoxins–research for environmental safety and human health. In: Chorus I, editor. Cyanotoxins–Occurence, Causes, Consequences. Springer-Verlag: Berlin; 2001. pp. 1-4

[8] Bláha L, Babica P, Maršálek B. Toxins produced in cyanobacterial water bloom–toxicity and risks. Interdisciplinary Toxicology. 2009;**2**(2):36-41

[9] Paerl HW, Huisman J. Climate change: A catalyst for global expansion of harmful cyanobacterial blooms. Environmental Microbiology. 2009;**1**:27-37

[10] Pantelić D, Svirčev Z, Simeunović J, Vidović M, Trajković I. Cyanotoxins: Characteristics, production and degradation routes in drinking water treatment with reference to the situation in Serbia. Chemosphere. 2013;**91**:421-441

[11] Svirčev Z, Lalić D, Bojadžija Savić G, Tokodi N, Drobac Backović D, Chen L, et al. Global geographical and historical overview of cyanotoxin distribution and cyanobacterial poisonings. Archives of Toxicology. 2019;**93**:2429-2248

[12] Briand JF, Jacquet S, Bernard C, Humbert JF. Health hazards for terrestrial vertebrates from toxic cyanobacteria in surface water ecosystems. Veterinary Research. 2003;**34**(4):361-377

[13] Falconer IR. Health effects associated with controlled exposures to cyanobacterial toxins. In: Hudnell KH, editor. Cyanobacterial Harmful Algal Blooms: State of the Science and Research Needs. New York: Springer; 2008. pp. 607-612

[14] Kuiper-Goodman T, Falconer IR, Fitzgerald J. Human health aspects. In: Chorus I, Bartram J, editors. Toxic Cyanobacteria in Water: A Guide to their Public Health Consequences, Monitoring and Management. London: E & FN Spon; 1999. pp. 113-153

[15] Svirčev V, Krstić S, Miladinov-Mikov M, Baltić V, Vidović M. Freshwater cyanobacterial blooms and primary liver cancer

epidemiological studies in Serbia. Journal of Environmental Science and Health. 2009;**C 27**:36-55

[16] Matsunaga H, Harada KI, Senma M, Ito Y, Yasuda N, Ushida S, et al. Possible cause of unnatural mass death of wild birds in a pond in Nishinomiya, Japan: Sudden appearance of toxic cyanobacteria. Natural Toxins. 1999;7(2):81-84

[17] Jochimsen EM, Carmichael WW, An J, Cardo DM, Cookson ST, Holmes CEM, et al. Liver failure and death after exposure to microcystins at a haemodialysis center in Brazil. The New England Journal of Medicine. 1998;**338**(13):873-878

[18] Pouria S, Andrade A, Barbosa J, Cavalcanti RL, Barreto VT, Ward CJ, et al. Fatal microcystin intoxication in haernodialysis unit in Caruaru, Brazil. Lancet. 1998;**352**:21-26

[19] Singh NK, Dhar DW. Cyanotoxins, related health hazards on animals and their management: A review. The Indian Journal of Animal Sciences. 2013;**83**:1111-1127

[20] Chiswell RK, Shaw GR, Eaglesham GK, Smith MJ, Norris RL, Seawright AA, et al. Stability of cylindrospermopsin, the toxin from the cyanobacterium *Cylindrospermopsis raciborskii*: Effects of pH, temperature and sunlight on decomposition. Environmental Toxicology. 1999;**14**:155-161

[21] Codd GA. Cyanobacterial toxins, the perception of water quality, and the prioritisation of eutrophication control. Ecological Engineering. 2000;**16**:51-60

[22] Ibelings BW, Chorus I. Accumulation of cyanobacterial toxins in freshwater "seafood" and its consequences for public health: A review. Environmental Pollutant. 2007;**150**:177-192

[23] Ettoumi A, El Khalloufi F, El Ghazali I, Oudra B, Amrani A, Nasri H, et al. Bioaccumulation of cyanobacterial toxins in aquatic organisms and its consequences for public health. In: Kattel G, editor. Zooplankton and Phyto-Plankton: Types, Characteristics and Ecology. New York: Nova Science Publishers Inc; 2011. pp. 1-34

[24] Hereman TC, Bittencourt-Oliveira MDC. Bioaccumulation of microcystins in lettuce. Journal of Phycology. 2012;**48**(6):1535-1537

[25] Anderson DM, Kaoru Y, White AW. Estimated Annual Economic Impacts from Harmful Algal Blooms (HABs) in United States. Woods Hole Oceanographic Institute Technical Report. Woods Hole Oceanographic Institution; 2000. DOI: 10.1575/1912/96

[26] Babica P, Blaha L, Marsalek B. Exploring the natural role of microcystins—A review of effects on photoautotrophic organisms. Journal of Phycology. 2006;**42**(1):9-20

[27] Weirich CA, Miller TR. Freshwater harmful algal blooms: Toxins and children's health. Current Problems in Pediatric and Adolescent Health Care. 2014;**44**:2-24

[28] Lopez CB, Jewett EB, Dortch Q, Walton BT, Hudnell HK. Scientific Assessment of Freshwater Harmful Algal Blooms. Washington, DC: Interagency Working Group on Harmful Algal Blooms, Hypoxia, and Human Health of the Joint Subcommittee on Ocean Science and Technology; 2008. p. 62. Available from: http://hdl.handle.net/1834/30786

[29] Moore RE. Public health and toxins from marine blue-green algae. In:

Ragelis EP, editor. Seafood Toxins. ACS Symposium Series No. 262. Washington: American Chemical Society; 1984. pp. 369-376

[30] Ressom R, Soong FS, Fitzgerald J, Turczynowicz L, El Saadi O, Roder D, et al. Health Effects of Toxic Cyanobacteria (Blue-Green Algae). Australian National Health and Medical Research Council, Looking Glass Press. Adelaide: University of Adelaide: South Australian Health Commission; 1993. pp. 67-90. ISBN: 9780730822752

[31] Hitzfeld BC, Höger SJ, Dietrich DR. Cyanobacterial toxins: Removal during drinking water treatment, and human risk assessment. Environmental Health Perspectives. 2000;**108**:113-122

[32] Cox PA, Banack SA, Murch SJ. Biomagnification of cyanobacterial neurotoxins and neurodegenerative disease among the Chamorro people of Guam. Proceedings of the National Academy of Sciences of the United States of America. 2003;**100**(23):13380-13383

[33] Metcalf JS, Richer R, Cox PA, Codd GA. Cyanotoxins in desert environments may present a risk to human health. Science of the Total Environment. 2012;**421-422**:118-123

[34] Kurki-Helasmo K, Meriluoto J. Microcystin uptake inhibits growth and protein phosphatase activity in mustard (*Sinapis alba* L.) seedlings. Toxicon. 1998;**36**:1921-1926

[35] McElhiney J, Lawton LA, Leifert C. Investigations into the inhibitory effects of microcystins on plant growth, and the toxicity of plant tissues following exposure. Toxicon. 2001;**39**:1411-1420

[36] Drobac D, Tokodi N, Kiprovski B, Malenčić D, Važić T, Nybom S, et al. Microcystin accumulation and potential effects on antioxidant capacity of leaves and fruits of *Capsicum annuum*. Journal of Toxicology and Environmental Health. 2017;**80**:145-154

[37] Carmichael WW. Cyanobacteria secondary metabolites—The cyanotoxins. The Journal of Applied Bacteriology. 1992;**72**:445-459

[38] Sivonen K, Jones G. Cyanobacterial toxins. In: Chorus I, Bartram J, editors. Toxic Cyanobacteria in Water: A Guide to Public Health Significance, Monitoring and Management. London: E&FN Spon; 1999. pp. 41-111

[39] Corbel S, Mougin C, Bouaïcha N. Cyanobacterial toxins: Modes of actions, fate in aquatic and soil ecosystems, phytotoxicity and bioaccumulation in agricultural crops. Chemosphere. 2014;**96**:1-15

[40] Sanchez JA, Otero P, Alfonso A, Ramos V, Vasconcelos V, Aráoz R, et al. Detection of anatoxin-a and three analogs in *Anabaena* spp. cultures: New fluorescence polarization assay and toxin profile by LC-MS/MS. Toxins. 2014;**6**:402-415

[41] Carmichael WW. The cyanotoxins. In: Callow JA, editor. Advances in Botanical Research, 47. London: Academic Press; 1997. pp. 211-255

[42] Sarma TA. Cyanobacterial toxins. In: Handbook of Cyanobacteria. Boca Raton, Florida: CRC Press, Taylor and Francis Group; 2013. pp. 487-606

[43] Krishnamurthy T, Carmichael WW, Sarver EW. Toxic peptides from freshwater cyanobacteria (blue-green algae) I. Isolation, purification and characterization of peptides from *Microcystis aeruginosa* and *Anabaena flos-aquae*. Toxicon. 1986;**24**:865-873

[44] Sivonen K, Namikoshi M, Evans WR, Carmichael WW, Sun F, Rouhiainen L, et al. Isolation and characterization of a variety of microcystins from seven strains of the cyanobacterial genus *Anabaena*. Applied Environmental Microbiology. 1992;**58**:2495-2500

[45] Fischer WJ, Altheimer S, Cattori V, Meier PJ, Dietrich DR, Hagenbuch B. Organic anion transporting polypeptides expressed in liver and brain mediate uptake of microcystin. Toxicology and Applied Pharmacology. 2005;**203**:257-263

[46] Chen L, Chen J, Zhang X, Xie P. A review of reproductive toxicity of microcystins. Journal of Hazardous Materials. 2015;**301**:381-399

[47] Eriksson JE, Toivola D, Meriluoto JAO, Karaki HYG, Hartshome D. Hepatocyte deformation induced by cyanobacterial toxins reflects inhibition of protein phosphatases. Biochemical and Biophysical Research Communications. 1990;**173**:1347-1352

[48] Matsushima R, Yoshizawa S, Watanabe MF, Harada K, Furusawa M, Carmichael WW, et al. In vitro and in vivo effects of protein phosphatase inhibitors, microcystins and nodularin, on mouse skin and fibroblasts. Biochemical and Biophysical Research Communications. 1990;**171**:867-874

[49] Yoshizawa S, Matsushima R, Watanabe MF, Harada K-I, Ichihara A, Carmichael WW, et al. Inhibition of protein phosphatases by microcystins and nodularin associated with hepatoxicity. Journal of Cancer Research and Clinical Oncology. 1990;**116**:609-614

[50] Toivola DM, Eriksson JE, Brautigar DL. Identification of protein phosphatase 2A as the primary target for microcystin-LR in rat liver homogenates. FEBS Letters. 1994;**344**:175-180

[51] Spoof L, Catherine A. Appendices 3. Tables of microcystins and nodularins. In: Meriluoto J, Spoof L, Codd GA, editors. Handbook of Cyanobacterial Monitoring and Cyanotoxin Analysis. John Wiley & Sons, Ltd; 2017. p. 576. ISBN: 978-1-119-06868-6

[52] de la Cruz AA, Antoniou MG, Hiskia A, Pelaez M, Song W, O'Shea KE, et al. Can we effectively degrade microcystins? Implications on human health. Anti-Cancer Agents in Medical Chemistry. 2011;**11**:19-37

[53] Fawell JK, James CP, James HA. Toxins from Blue-Green Algae: Toxicological Assessment of Microcystin-LR and a Method for its Determination in Water. Medmenham, UK: Water Research Centre; 1994. pp. 1-46

[54] Mahakhant A, Sano T, Ratanachot P, Tongaram T, Srivastava VC, Watanabe MM, et al. Detection of microcystins from cyanobacterial water blooms in Thailand fresh water. Phycology Research. 1998;**42**:25-29. DOI: 10.1046/j.1440-1835.1998.00119.x

[55] Vieira JM d S, Azevedo MT d P, SMF d OA, Honda RY, Corrêa B. Microcystin production by *Radiocystisfernandoi* (*Chroococcales*, *cyanobacteria*) isolated from a drinking water reservoir in the city of Belém, PA, Brazilian Amazonia region. Toxicon. 2003;**42**:709-713

[56] Ballot A. Cyanobacteria and cyanobacterial toxins in three alkaline Rift Valley lakes of Kenya--Lakes Bogoria, Nakuru and Elmenteita. Journal of Plankton Research. 2004;**26**:925-935. DOI: 10.1093/plankt/fbh084

[57] Ballot A, Krienitz L, Kotut K, Wiegand C, Pflugmacher S.

Cyanobacteria and cyanobacterial toxins in the alkaline crater lakes Sonachi and Simbi, Kenya. Harmful Algae. 2005;**4**:139-150. DOI: 10.1016/j.hal.2004.01.001

[58] Fiore MF, Genuário DB, da Silva CSP, Shishido TK, Moraes LAB, CantúsioNeto R, et al. Microcystin production by a freshwater spring cyanobacterium of the genus *Fischerella*. Toxicon. 2009;**53**:754-761. DOI: 10.1016/j.toxicon.2009.02.010

[59] Sivonen K, Kononen K, Carmichael WW, Dahlem AM, Rinehart KL, Kiviranta J, et al. Occurrence of the hepatotoxic cyanobacterium *Nodularia spumigena* in the Baltic Sea and structure of the toxin. Applied and Environmental Microbiology. 1989;**55**:1990-1995

[60] Carmichael WW, Boyer GL. Health impacts from cyanobacteria harmful algae blooms: Implications for the north American Great Lakes. Harmful Algae. 2016;**54**:194-212

[61] Ohtani I, Moore RE, Runnegar MTC. Cylindrospermopsin: A potent hepatotoxin from the blue-green alga *Cylindrospermopsis raciborskii*. Journal of the American Chemical Society. 1992;**114**(20):7941-7942

[62] Li R, Carmichael WW, Brittain S, Eaglesham GK, Shaw GR, Watanabe MM. First report of the cyanotoxins cylindrospermopsin and deoxycylindrospermopsin from *Raphidiopsis curvata* (cyanobacteria). Journal of Phycology. 2001;**37**:1121-1126

[63] Schembri MA, Neilan BA, Saint CP. Identification of genes implicated in toxin production in the cyanobacterium *Cylindrospermopsis raciborskii*. Environmental Toxicology. 2001;**16**:413-421

[64] Svrcek C, Smith DW. Cyanobacteria toxins and the current state of knowledge on water treatment options: A review. Journal of Environmental Engineering and Science. 2004;**3**(3):155-185

[65] Spoof L, Berg KA, Rapala J, Lahti K, Lepisto L, Metcalf JS, et al. First observation of cylindrospermopsin in *Anabaena lapponica* isolated from the boreal environment (Finland). Environmental Toxicology. 2006;**21**:552-560

[66] Seifert M, McGregor G, Eaglesham G, Wickramasinghe W, Shaw G. First evidence for the production of cylindrospermopsin and deoxy-cylindrosper-mopsin by the freshwater benthic cyanobacterium, *Lyngbya wollei* (Farlow ex Gornont) Speziale and Dyck. Harmful Algae. 2007;**6**(1):73-80

[67] Devlin JP, Edwards OE, Gorham PR, Hunter MR, Pike RK, Stavric B. Anatoxin-a, a toxic alkaloid from *Anabaena flosaquae* NCR-44h. The Canadian Journal of Chemistry. 1977;**55**:1367-1371

[68] Carmichael WW, Gorham P. Anatoxins from clones of *Anabaena flos-aquae* isolated from lakes of Western Canada. Mitteilung Internationale Vereinigung fuer Limnologie. 1978;**21**:285-295

[69] Fitzgeorge RB, Clark SA, Keevil CW. Routes of intoxication. In: Codd GA, Jefferies TM, Keevil CW, Potter E, editors. Detection Methods for Cyanobacterial Toxins. Cambridge: The Royal Society of Chemistry; 1994. pp. 69-74

[70] Van Apeldoorn ME, Van Egmond HP, Speijers GJA, Bakker GJI. Toxins of cyanobacteria. Molecular Nutrition and Food Research. 2007;**51**(1):7-60

[71] Shams S, Capelli C, Cerasino L, Ballot A. Anatoxin-a producing *Tychonema* (cyanobacteria) in European waterbodies. Water Research. 2015;**69**:68-79

[72] Skulberg OM, Carmichael WW, Andersen RA, Matsunuga S, Moore RE, Skulberg R. Investigations of a neurotoxic oscillatorian strain (*Cyanophyceae*) and its toxin. Isolation and characterization of homoanatoxin-a. Environmental Toxicology Chemistry. 1992;**11**:321-329

[73] Codd GA, Ward CJ, Bell SG. Cyanobacterial toxins: Occurrence, modes of action, health effects and exposure routes. Archives of Toxicology Supplement. 1997;**19**:399-410

[74] Namikoshi M, Murakami T, Watanabe MF, Oda T, Yamada J, Tsujimura S, et al. Simultaneous production of homoanatoxin-a, anatoxin-a, and a new non-toxic 4-hydroxyhomoanatoxin-a by the cyanobacterium *Raphidiopsis mediterranea* Skuja. Toxicon. 2003;**42**:533-538

[75] Mahmood WA, Carmichael WW. Anatoxin-a(s), an anticholinesterase from the cyanobacterium *Anabaena flos-aquae* NRC- 525-17. Toxicon. 1987;**25**:1211-1227

[76] Matsunaga S, Moore RE, Niemczura WP, Carmichael WW. Anatoxin-a(s), a potent anticholinesterase from *Anabaena flos-aquae*. Journal of the American Chemical Society. 1989;**111**:8021-8023

[77] Carmichael WW, Mahmood NA, Hyde EG. Natural toxins from cyanobacteria (blue-green algae). In: Hall S, Strichartz G, editors. Marine Toxins: Origin, Structure, and Molecular Pharmacology. Washington DC: American Chemical Society; 1990. pp. 87-106

[78] Stewart I. Recreational Exposure to Freshwater Cyanobacteria: Epidemiology, Dermal Toxicity and Biological Activity of Cyanobacterial Lipopolysaccharides. [Thesis]. School of Population Health, University of Queensland; 2004. pp. 1-418

[79] Aráoz R, Molgó J, Tandeau de Marsac N. Neurotoxic cyanobacterial toxins. Toxicon. 2010;**56**(5):813-828

[80] Humpage AR, Rositano J, Breitag AH, Brown R, Baler PD, Nicholson WC, et al. Paralytic shellfish poisons from Australian cyanobacterial blooms. Australian Journal of Marine and Freshwater Research. 1994;**45**:761-777

[81] Mons MN, Van Egmond HP, Speijers GJA. Paralytic Shellfish Poisoning: A Review. Bilthoven, The Netherlands: RIVM; 1998. p. 60. 388802005

[82] Beltran EC, Neilan BA. Geographical segregation of the neurotoxin-producing cyanobacterium *Anabaena circinalis*. Applied Environmental Microbiology. 2000;**66**:4468-4474

[83] World Health Organization. Guidelines for Safe Recreational Water Environments. Volume 1, Coastal and Fresh Waters. World Health Organization; 2003. p. 33. ISBN 921545801

[84] Wiese M, D'Agostino PM, Mihali TK, Moffitt MC, Neilan BA. Neurotoxic alkaloids: Saxitoxin and its analogs. Marine Drugs. 2010;**8**(7):2185-2211

[85] Cirés S, Ballot A. A review of the phylogeny, ecology and toxin production of bloom-forming *Aphanizomenon* spp.

and related species within the *Nostocales* (cyanobacteria). Harmful Algae. 2016;**54**:21-43

[86] Cox PA, Banack SA, Murch SJ, Rasmussen U, Tien G, Bidigare RR, et al. Diverse taxa of cyanobacteria produce beta-N-methylamino-L-alanine, a neurotoxic amino acid. PNAS. 2005;**102**(14):5074-5078

[87] Fujiki H, Sugimura T, Moore RE. New classes of environmental tumor promoters: Indole alkaloids and polyacetates. Environmental Health Perspectives. 1983;**50**:85-90

[88] Ito E, Satake M, Yasumoto T. Pathological effects of lyngbyatoxin A upon mice. Toxicon. 2002;**40**:551-556

[89] Moore RE, Blackman AJ, Cheuk CE, Mynderse JS, Matsumoto GK, Clardy J, et al. Absolute stereochemistries of the aplysiatoxins and oscillatoxin A. Journal of Organic Chemistry. 1984;**49**:2484-2489

[90] Stewart I, Schluter PJ, Shaw GR. Cyanobacterial lipopolysaccharides and human health–a review. Environmental Health: A Global Access Science Source. 2006;**5**:7

[91] Chen Y, Shen D, Fang D. Nodularins in poisoning. Clinica Chimica Acta. 2013;**425**:18-29

[92] Boopathi T, Ki JS. Impact of environmental factors on the regulation of cyanotoxin production. Toxins (Basel.). 2014;**6**(7):1951-1978

[93] Botes DP, Kruger H, Viljoen CC. Isolation and characterization of four toxins from the blue-green alga microcystis aeruginosa. Toxicon. 1982;**20**:945-954

[94] Merel S, Clement M, Thomas O. State of the art on cyanotoxins in water and their behaviour towards chlorine. Toxicon. 2010;**55**:677-691

[95] Bouaïcha N, Maatouk I. Microcystin-LR and nodularin induce intracellular glutathione alteration, reactive oxygen species production and lipid peroxidation in primary cultured rat hepatocytes. Toxicology Letters. 2004;**148**:53-63

[96] Gehringer MM, Adler L, Roberts AA, Moffitt MC, Mihali TK, Mills TJT, et al. Nodularin, a cyanobacterial toxin, is synthesized in plants by symbiotic *Nostoc* sp. ISME Journal. 2012;**6**(10):1834-1847

[97] de la Cruz AA, Hiskia A, Kaloudis T, Chernoff N, Hill D, Antoniou MG, et al. A review on cylindrospermopsin: The global occurrence, detection, toxicity and degradation of a potent cyanotoxin. Environmental Science. Processes and Impacts. 2013;**15**(11):1979-2003

[98] Yang YM, Yu GL, Chen YX, Jia NN, Li RH. Four decades of progress in cylindrospermopsin research: The ins and outs of a potent cyanotoxin. Journal of Hazardous Materials. 2021;**406**:124653

[99] Hawkins PR, Chandrasena NR, Jones GJ, Humpage AR, Falconer IR. Isolation and toxicity of *Cylindrospermopsis raciborskii* from an ornamental lake. Toxicon. 1997;**35**:341-346

[100] Harada K-I, Ohtani I, Iwamoto K, Suzuki M, Watanabe MF, Watanabe M, et al. Isolation of cylindrospermopsin from a cyanobacterium Ume-zakia natans and its screening method. Toxicon. 1994;**32**(1):73-84

[101] Banker R, Carmeli S, Hadas O, Teltsch B, Porat R, Sukenik A. Identification of cylindrospermopsin in *Aphanizomenon ovalisporum* (Cyanophyceae) isolated from Lake

Kinneret, Israel. Journal of Phycolology. 1997;**33**(4):613-616

[102] Carmichael WW, Falconer IR. Diseases related to freshwater blue-green algal toxins and control measures. In: Falconer IR, editor. Algal Toxins in Seafood and Drinking Water. London: Academic Press; 1993. pp. 187-209

[103] Duy TN, Lam PKS, Shaw GR, Connell DW. Toxicology and risk assessment of freshwater cyanobacterial (blue-green algal) toxins in water. Reviews of Environmental Contamination and Toxicology. 2000;**163**:113-186

[104] Wiegand C, Pflugmacher S. Ecotoxicological effects of selected cyanobacterial secondary metabolites: A short review. Toxicology and Applied Pharmacology. 2005;**203**:201-218

[105] Mahmood NA, Carmichael WW. The pharmacology of anatoxin-a(s), a neurotoxin produced by the freshwater cyanobacterium *Anabaena flos-aquae* NRC 525-17. Toxicon. 1986;**24**:425-434

[106] Negri AP, Jones GJ. Bioaccumulation of paralytic shellfish poisoning (PSP) toxins from the cyanobacterium *Anabaena circinalis* by the freshwater mussel *Alathyriq condola*. Toxicon. 1995;**33**(5):667-678

[107] Carmichael WW, Evans WR, Yin QQ, Bell P, Moczydlowski E. Evidence for paralytic shellfish poisons in the freshwater cyanobacterium *Lyngbya wollei* (Farlow ex Gomont) comb.nov. Journal of Applied and Environmental Microbiology. 1997;**63**(8):3104-3110

[108] Onodera H, Oshima Y, Henriksen P, Yasumoto T. Confirmation of anatoxin–a(s), in the cyanobacterium *Anabaena lemmermannii*, as the cause of bird kills in Danish lakes. Toxicon. 1997;**35**(11):1645-1648

[109] Foss AJ, Phlips EJ, Yilmaz M, Chapman A. Characterization of paralytic shellfish toxins from *Lyngbya wollei* dominated mats collected from two Florida springs. Harmful Algae. 2012;**16**:98-107

[110] Carmichael WW. The toxins of cyanobacteria. Scientific American. 1994;**170**(1):78-86

[111] Carmichael WW, Biggs DF, Peterson MA. Pharmacology of anatoxin-a, produced by the freshwater cyanophyte *Anabaena flos-aquae* NRC-44-1. Toxicon. 1979;**17**:229-236

[112] Harada K, Kimura Y, Ogawa K, Suzuki M, Dahlem AM, Beasley VR, et al. A new procedure for the analysis and purification of naturally occurring anatoxin-a from the blue-green alga *Anabaena flos-aquae*. Toxicon. 1989;**27**:1289-1296

[113] Rantala-Ylinen A, Kana S, Wang H, Rouhiainen L, Wahlsten M, Rizzi E, et al. Anatoxin-a synthetase gene cluster of the cyanobacterium *Anabaena* sp. strain 37 and molecular methods to detect potential producers. Journal of Applied and Environmental Microbiology. 2011;**77**(20):7271-7278

[114] Selwood AI, Holland PT, Wood SA, Smith KF, McNabb PS. Production of anatoxin-a and a novel biosynthetic precursor by the cyanobacterium *Aphanizomenon issatschenkoi*. Environmental Science and Technology. 2007;**41**:506-510

[115] Ballot A, Fastner J, Wiedner C. Paralytic shellfish poisoning toxin-producing cyanobacterium *Aphanizomenon gracile* in Northeast

Germany. Applied and Environmental Microbiology. 2010;**76**(4):1173-1180

[116] Aráoz R, Nghiêm HO, Rippka R, Palibroda N, de Marsac NT, Herdman M. Neurotoxins in axenic oscillatorian cyanobacteria: Coexistence of anatoxin-a and homoanatoxin-a determined by ligand-binding assay and GC/MS. Micro-biology (Reading, Engl.). 2005;**151**:1263-1273

[117] Cadel-Six S, Peyraud-Thomas C, Brient L, de Marsac NT, Rippka R, Májean A. Different genotypes of anatoxin-producing cyanobacteria coexist in the Tarn river, France. Applied and Environmental Microbiology. 2007;**73**:7605-7614

[118] Viaggiu E, Melchiorre S, Volpi F, Di Corcia A, Mancini R, Garibaldi L, et al. Anatoxin-a toxin in the cyanobacterium *Planktothrix rubescens* from a fishing pond in northern Italy. Environmental Toxicology. 2004;**19**(3):191-197

[119] Park HD, Watanabe MF, Harda K, Nagai H, Suzuki M, Watanabe M, et al. Hepatotoxin (microcystin) and neurotoxin (anatoxin-a) contained in natural blooms and strains of cyanobacteria from Japanese freshwaters. Natural Toxins. 1993;**1**:353-360

[120] Ghassempour A, Najafi NM, Mehdinia A, Davarani SSH, Fallahi M, Nakhshab M. Analysis of anatoxin-a using polyaniline as a sorbent in solid-phase microextraction coupled to gas chromatography-mass spectrometry. Journal of Chromatography. A. 2005;**1078**:120-127

[121] Gugger M, Lenoir S, Berger C, Ledreux A, Druart JC, Humbert JF, et al. First report in a river in France of the benthic cyanobacterium *Phormidium favosum* producing anatoxin–a associated with dog neurotoxicosis. Toxicon. 2005;**45**(7):919-928

[122] Ballot A, Krienitz L, Kotut K, Wiegand C, Metcalf JS, Codd GA, et al. Cyanobacteria and cyanobacterial toxins in three alkaline Rift Valley lakes of Kenya—Lakes Bogoria, Nakuru and Elmenteita. Journal of Plankton Research. 2004;**26**:925-935

[123] Méjean A, Peyraud-Thomas C, Kerbrat AS, Golubic S, Pauillac S, Chinain M, et al. First identification of the neurotoxin homoanatoxin-a from mats of *Hydrocoleum lyngbyaceum* (marine cyanobacterium) possibly linked to giant clam poisoning in New Caledonia. Toxicon. 2010;**56**:829-835

[124] Wood SA, Rasmussen JP, Holland PT, Campbell R, Crowe ALM. First report of the cyanotoxin anatoxin-a from *Aphanizomenon issatschenkoi* (cyanobacteria). Journal of Phycology. 2007;**43**(2):356-365

[125] Ballot A, Fastner J, Lentz M, Wiedner C. First report of anatoxin-a-producing cyanobacterium *Aphanizomenon issatschenkoi* in northeastern Germany. Toxicon. 2010;**56**(6):964-971

[126] Jiang Y, Song G, Pan Q, Yang Y, Li R. Identification of genes for anatoxin-a biosynthesis in *Cuspidothrix issatschenkoi*. Harmful Algae. 2015;**46**:43-48

[127] Gorham PR, Carmichael WW. Hazards of freshwater blue-green algae (cyanobacteria). In: Lembi AA, Waaland JR, editors. Algae and Human Affairs. Cambridge: Cambridge University Press; 1988. pp. 403-431

[128] Weise G, Drews G, Jann B, Jann K. Identification and analysis of a lipopolysaccharide in cell walls of the

blue-green algae *Anacystis nidulans*. Archives of Microbiology. 1970;**71**:89-98

[129] Codd GA, Morrison LF, Metcalf JS. Cyanobacterial toxins: Risk management for health protection. Toxicology and Applied Pharmacology. 2005;**203**:264-272

[130] Weckesser J, Drews G. Lipopolysaccharides of photosynthetic prokaryotes. In: Chorus I, Bartram J, editors. Toxic Cyanobacteria in Water: A Guide to their Public Health Consequences, Monitoring and Management. London and New York: E & FN Spon. An Imprint of Routledge; 1979. pp. 215-239

[131] Taylor MS, Stahl-Timmins W, Redshaw CH, Osborne NJ. Toxic alkaloids in *Lyngbya majuscula* and related tropical marine cyanobacteria. Harmful Algae. 2014;**31**:1-8

[132] Jiang W, Zhou W, Uchida H, Kikumori M, Irie K, Watanabe R, et al. A new lyngbyatoxin from the Hawaiian cyanobacterium *Moorea* producens. Marine Drugs. 2014;**12**(5):2748-2759

[133] Chlipala GE, Tri PH, Hung NV, Krunić A, Shim SH, Soejarto DD, et al. Nhatrangins A and B, aplysiatoxin-related metabolites from the marine cyanobacterium *Lyngbya majuscula* from Vietnam. Journal of Natural Products. 2010;**73**(4):784-787

[134] Gupta D, Kaur P, Leong S, Tan L, Prinsep M, Chu J. Anti-chikungunya viral activities of aplysiatoxin-related compounds from the marine cyanobac-terium *Trichodesmium erythraeum*. Marine Drugs. 2014;**12**(1):115-127

[135] Raziuddin S, Siegelman HW, Tornabene TG. Lipopolysaccharides of the cyanobacterium *Microcystis aeruginosa*. European Journal of Biochemistry. 1983;**137**:333-336

[136] Banack SA, Johnson HE, Cheng R, Cox PA. Production of neurotoxic BMAA by marine cyanobacteria. Marine Drugs. 2007;**5**:180-196

[137] Spencer PS, Nunn PB, Hugon J, Ludolph AC, Ross SM, Roy DN, et al. Guam amyotrophic lateral sclerosis—Parkinsonism–dementia linked to a plant excitant neurotoxin. Science. 1987;**237**(4814):517-522

[138] Garamszegi SP, Banack SA, Duque LL, Metcalf JS, EWl S, Cox PA, et al. Detection of β-N-methylamino-l-alanine in postmortem olfactory bulbs of Alzheimer's disease patients using UHPLC-MS/MS: An autopsy case-series study. Toxicology Reports. 2023;**10**:87-96

[139] Falconer IR. Potential impact on human health of toxic cyanobacteria. Phycologia. 1996;**35**:6-11

[140] Falconer IR. Is there a human health hazard from microcystins in the drinking water supply? Acta Hydrochimica et Hydrobiologica. 2005;**33**(1):64-71

[141] Eriksson JE, Meriluoto J, Lindholm T. Accumulation of a peptide toxin from the cyanobacterium *Oscillatoria agardhii* in the freshwater mussel *Anodonta cygnea*. Hydrobiology. 1989;**183**:211-216

[142] Ferrão-Filho AS. Bioacumulação de cianotoxinas e seus efeitos em organismos aquáticos. Oecologia Australis. 2009;**13**(2):272-312

[143] Gilroy DJ, Kauffman KW, Hall RA, Huang X, Chu FS. Assessing potential health risks from microcystin toxins in blue-green algae dietary supplements. Environmental Health Perspectives. 2000;**108**:435-439

[144] Pilotto LS, Douglas RM, Burch MD, Cameron S, Beers M, Rouch GR, et al. Health effects of recreational exposure to cyanobacteria (blue-green algae) during recreational water-related activities. Australian and New Zealand Journal of Public Health. 1997;**21**:562-566

[145] Wood SA, Dietrich DR. Quantitative assessment of aerosolized cyanobacterial toxins at two New Zealand lakes. Journal of Environmental Monitoring. 2011;**13**(6):1617-1624

[146] Metcalf JS, Banack SA, Richer R, Cox PA. Neurotoxic aminoacids and their isomers in desert environments. Journal of Arid Environment. 2015;**112**:140-144

[147] Codd GA, Bell S, Kaya K, Ward C, Beattie K, Metcalf J. Cyanobacterial toxins, exposure routes and human health. European Journal of Phycology. 1999;**34**(4):405-415

[148] Azevedo SM, Carmichael WW, Jochimsen EM, Rinehart KL, Lau S, Shaw GR, et al. Human intoxication by microcystins during renal dialysis treatment in Caruaru-Brazil. Toxicology. 2002;**181**:441-446

[149] Mohamed ZA, Elnour RO, Alamri S, et al. Occurrence of β-N-methylamino-L-alanine (BMAA) toxin in irrigation water and field vegetable plants and assessing its potential risk to human health. Water, Air, and Soil Pollution. 2024;**235**:72. DOI: 10.1007/s11270-023-06861-0

[150] Mohamed ZA, Elnour RO, Alamri S, et al. Presence of the neurotoxin β-N-methylamino-L-alanine in irrigation water and accumulation in cereal grains with human exposure risk. Environmental Science and Pollution Research. 2024;**31**(21):31479-31491. DOI: 10.1007/s11356-024-33188-y

[151] Bowling L. The Cyanobacterial (Blue-Green Algal) Bloom in the Darling/Barwon River System, November–December 1991. Sydney: NSW Department of Water Resources, Technical Services Division. Report No. 92; 1992. p. 074

[152] Pereira P, Onodera H, Andrinolo D, Franca S, Araujo F, Lagos N, et al. Paralytic shellfish toxins in the freshwater cyanobacterium *Aphanizomenon flos-aquae*, isolated from Montargil reservoir, Portugal. Toxicon. 2000;**38**:1689-1702

[153] Carmichael WW, Azevedo SM, An JS, Molica RJ, Jochimsen EM, Lau S, et al. Human fatalities from cyanobacteria: Chemical and biological evidence for cyanotoxins. Environmental Health Perspectives. 2001;**109**:663-668

[154] Hindman SH, Favero MS, Carson LA, Petersen NJ, Schonberger LB, Solano JT. Pyrogenic reactions during haemodialysis caused by extramural endotoxin. The Lancet. 1975;**2**:732-734

[155] Metcalf JS, Codd GA. Cyanobacterial Toxins (Cyanotoxins) in Water. Marlow, Bucks SL 7 1FD, U.K.: Foundation for water research Allen House, The Listons, Liston Road; 2004

[156] Teixera M, Costa M, Carvalho V, Pereira M, Hage E. Gastroenteritis epidemic in the area of the Itaparica Dam, Bahia, Brazil. Bulletin of the Pan American Health Organiyation. 1993;**27**:244-253

[157] Drobac D, Svirčev Z, Tokodi N, Vidović M, Baltić V, Božić-Krstić V, et al. Microcystins—Potential risk factors in carcinogenesis of primary liver cancer in Serbia. Geographica Pannonica. 2011;**15**:70-80

[158] Cox PA, Kostrzewa RM, Guillemin GJ. BMAA and neurodegenerative illness. Neurotoxicity Research. 2018;**33**:178-183. DOI: 10.1007/s12640-017-9753-6

[159] Zanchett G, Oliveira-Filho EC. Cyanobacteria and cyanotoxins: From impacts on aquatic ecosystems and human health to anticarcinogenic effects. Toxins. 2013;**5**:1896-1917

[160] Harada K, Oshikata M, Uchikata H, Suzuki M, Kondo F, Sato K, et al. Detection and identification of microcystin in the drinking water of Haimen city, China. Natural Toxins. 1996;**4**:277-283

[161] Zhou L, Yu H, Chen K. Relationship between microcystin in drinking water and colorectal cancer. Biomedical and Environmental Science. 2002;**15**(2):166-171

[162] Hernandez BY, Zhu X, Nagata M, Loo L, Chan O, Wong LL. Cyanotoxin exposure and hepatocellular carcinoma. Toxicology. 2023;**487**:153470

Chapter 7

Cyanobacterial Toxins: Our Line of Defense

Dijana Lalić

Abstract

Cyanobacteria (blue-green algae) are a diverse group of photo-autotrophic organisms where their higher dominance, in favorable conditions, represents a significant indicator of water quality. Some of the cyanobacterial genera are toxigenic and can produce toxins—cyanotoxins, which influence animals and humans' health, and also plants. Commonly known and studded cyanotoxin groups include hepatotoxins (microcystins, nodularins), cytotoxins (cylindrospermopsin), neurotoxins (saxitoxins, anatoxins, BMAA), dermatotoxins (lyngbyatoxin), and irritant toxins (lipopolysaccharide endotoxins). This chapter provides guideline values for the cyanotoxins in drinking water supply and in water for recreational purposes. This chapter focuses on a critical evaluation of the efficacy of water treatment procedures essential for cyanotoxin control. Such knowledge is extremely important in the future expansion of cyanobacterial toxic compounds from aquatic ecosystems, and according to the newest data, from terrestrial environments, especially due to climate change (global warming) and anthropogenic eutrophication. Here are introduced schemes of cyanobacterial ecology and infiltration of cyanotoxins through the biological cycle jeopardizing human health, and tables of the drinking water treatment, along with proposed therapy and limitations, setting the strong foundation for all future research, which are of outstanding scientific importance.

Keywords: cyanobacteria, cyanotoxins, toxicity, therapy, drinking water, cyanotoxins guideline values

1. Introduction

Cyanobacteria, also known as blue-green algae, are among the oldest known organisms on Earth, with fossils dating back over 3.5 billion years. Cyanobacteria are found in a wide range of habitats, including oceans, freshwater lakes, loess and desert crust, and even Antarctic rocks [1]. These groups are credited with producing a significant portion of the Earth's oxygen through photosynthesis. Some species of cyanobacteria can "fix" atmospheric nitrogen into a form that plants can use, playing a crucial role in the nitrogen cycle. Cyanobacteria contain a variety of secondary metabolites—pigments (phycocyanin, phycoerythrin, and allophycocyanin), that give them their characteristic blue-green color [1]; UV sunscreen pigments (scytonemin and mycosporine-like amino acids) and toxins (cyanotoxins), which enable them to thrive in diverse environments [1, 2]. Normally, algae are barely visible. Under favorable conditions, this can change as they rapidly increase in size to form large areas of greenish, floating scum on the surface water—cyanobacterial blooms. The incidence of cyanobacterial blooms in freshwaters has increased worldwide in the past decade, and they are one of the main problems that endanger the ecological function of water bodies [3] and now have been considered a global environmental public health issue [3–5]. Most algal blooms are natural and essential components of any water bodies, and most are non-toxic, however, certain cyanobacteria can produce cyanotoxins, cause foul smell (geosmin and methylisoborneol), and unaesthetic challenges to the environment [6]. The most common toxic cyanobacteria in freshwater are *Microcystis* spp., *Planktothrix rubescens*, *Raphidiopsis raciborskii* (formerly *Cylindrospermopsis raciborskii*), *Nostoc* spp., *Oscillatoria* spp., *Schizothrix* spp., and *Synechocystis* spp. [7]. During a cyanobacteria bloom, an excess of dead and decaying cyanobacteria can result in hypoxia or anoxia, resulting in fish kills mortality of fauna, and loss of flora [8, 9].

Cyanobacterial favorable conditions are applied to environmental conditions (bright sunlight, high nutrient levels, calm waters (low wind and circulation), limited number of grazers or predators, temperature and pH) and further, trace metals (such as iron, zinc, copper, and magnesium) and environmental pollutants [10]. Temperature higher than 20°C, with nutrients, promotes mineralization leading to explosive growth of cyanobacteria [9, 11], and leads to increased toxin release [12, 13]. pH promotes the proliferation of cyanobacteria, hence the production of cyanotoxins [14, 15]. Increases in nitrate concentration increased MCs production [16], and a deficiency of trace metals in water bodies stimulates the production of intracellular cyanotoxins to acquire or store these metals [17]. On the contrary, in the situation of high levels of trace metal, cyanobacteria produce extracellular toxins to create metal complexes and detoxify the metals [18]. Sources of nutrients can be from fertilizers in the farm during storm runoff [19] and from organisms or particles within the mat [20]. Their occurrence is most common in shallow waters [6].

Climate change has become a global trend, with warming at an unprecedented rate [21] being one of its most prominent manifestations. A global increase of industrialization and urbanization increased nutrient inputs by industrial wastewaters, agricultural runoff (fertilizer), animal waste, the flux of sewage, and detergent usage—eutrophication [3, 22]. The recent trend of climate warming and declining wind speeds has enhanced algal nitrogen and phosphorus utilization efficiency. The precipitation could affect terrestrial discharge, which possibly brings external nitrogen and phosphorus from the watershed into lakes [23, 24]. This can, as a cumulative reaction, enhance expansive cyanobacterial growth [9, 25–28]. In developing countries and rural areas, surface water bodies are under severe threat due to the uncontrolled disposal of industrial waste and the application of fertilizers on agricultural lands located near water bodies. Combined effects of eutrophication and climate change have increased the occurrence and intensity of cyanobacterial blooms, causing problems in aquatic ecosystems intended for drinking purposes and recreational use [3]. These increases are linked to the deterioration of water quality and increased threats to human sustainable development, social and economic welfare, and, most importantly, health (**Figure 1**).

So, it can be concluded that the occurrence of cyanobacteria in surface water bodies is usually a function of climate change (elevated warm temperature), soil erosion from agricultural fields, and eutrophication, dominantly caused by human activities. As a result, water resources for drinking and recreation purposes are

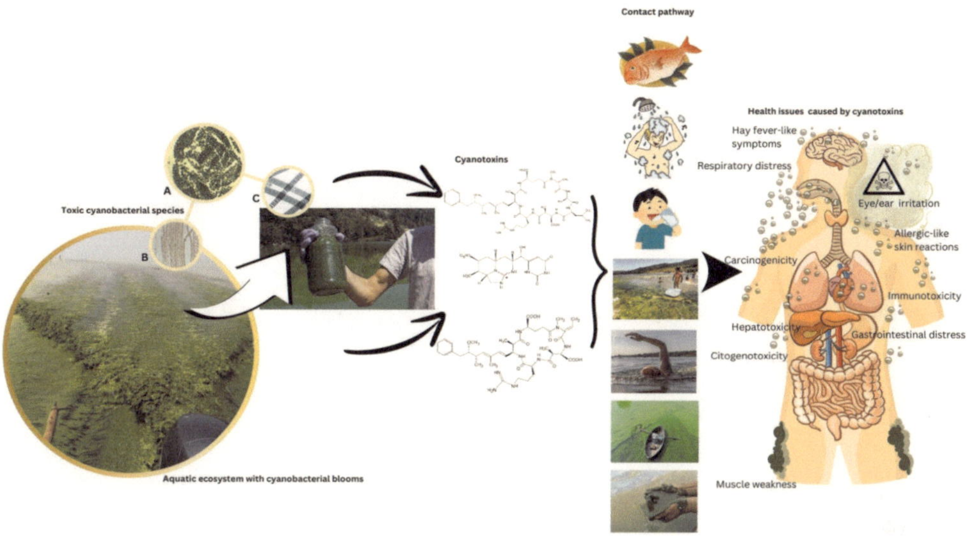

Figure 1.
Cyanobacterial blooms in the environment with toxic cyanobacterial species. (A) Microcystis aeruginosa*; (B)* Aphanizomenon flos-aquae*; (C)* Oscillatoria *sp. (Created by Author using Canva).*

adversely affected. The increasing trend of cyanobacterial blooms and associated toxin production will likely continue in the upcoming years [29, 30]. Therefore, it is important to introduce regular testing of water bodies for the presence of cyanobacteria and cyanotoxins to protect human health.

2. Cyanotoxins

2.1 Characteristics

Cyanobacteria are recognized as producers of a diverse range of secondary metabolites, where 50% of them are known to produce extremely toxic cyanotoxins. Cyanotoxins can be produced widely along with cyanobacterial blooms in the world [2]. The most commonly found cyanotoxins in freshwater bodies are microcystin, nodularin, cylindrospermopsin, anatoxin, guanitoxin (formerly known as anatoxin-a(S)), saxitoxin, lyngbyatoxins, and BMAA. There are over 300 different congeners of microcystins identified to date [31], and one of the most investigated and commonly found is microcystin-LR (MC-LR). CYN is the second most frequently reported cyanotoxin due to negative health effects in humans [32]. Cyanotoxins are a very diverse group of chemicals found in water for irrigation, recreation, and, most importantly, in water for drinking supplies. Cyanotoxins can be very potent and their production may threaten the health of humans and animals [2, 22, 33]. Cyanotoxins can be grouped based on their modes of action and target organs into hepatotoxins, neurotoxins, dermatotoxins, and cytotoxins [34], or based on their chemical structures into alkaloids, organophosphorus, cyclic peptides, and lipopolysaccharides compounds [35].

During the occurrence of cyanobacterial blooms, it is necessary to take caution about water-related activity (**Figure 2**). Some cyanotoxins have toxicities that are

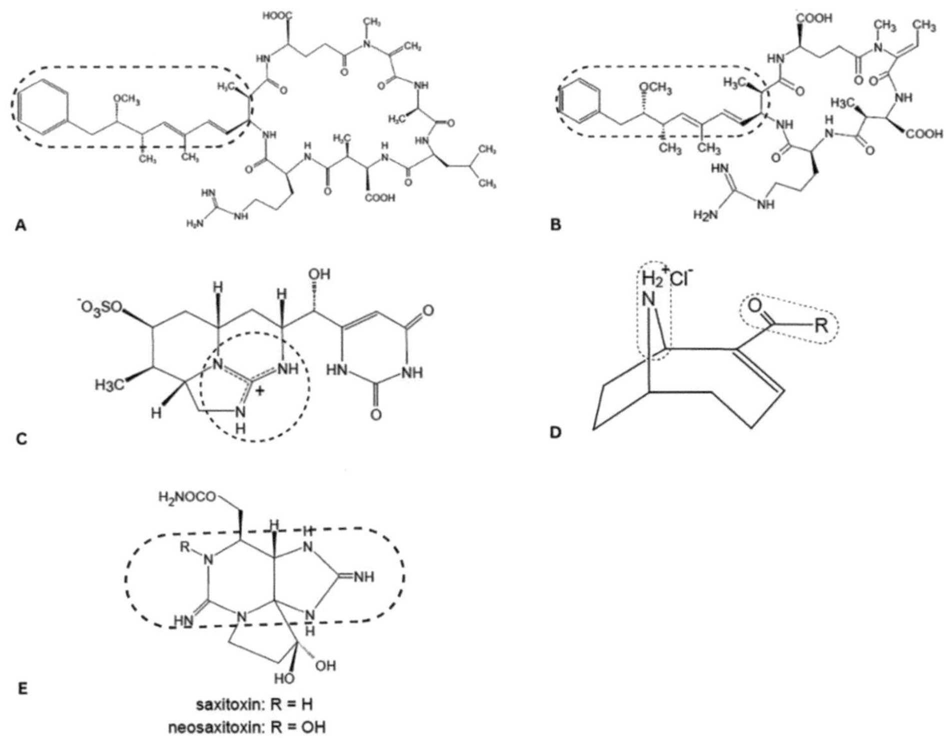

Figure 2.
Chemical structure of cyanotoxins. (Dashed area indicates the moiety most responsible for the cyanotoxin toxicity). (A) MC-LR; (B) NOD; (C) CYN; (D) ATX; (E) STX (Created by Author using ChemSketch).

comparable to, or in some cases more potent than, cyanide [3]. The presence of high levels of cyanotoxins in recreational and drinking water may cause a wide range of symptoms such as nausea, vomiting, salivation, incontinence, abdominal pain and diarrhea, headache, fever, skin rashes, muscle tremors, paralysis, respiratory failure, and even death in severe cases. These symptoms can occur in a couple of minutes to days after exposure. Also, they can cause damage to kidney and liver tissues [36]. Chronic effects of cyanotoxins cannot be neglected. Cyanobacteria may be present in water bodies over extended periods, which results in continued exposure to subacute concentrations, leading to the possibility of chronic health effects and possible carcinogenic changes [37–39]. While the severity of the effects can vary depending on the amount of the cyanotoxin, duration, and frequency of exposure, susceptibility to cyanotoxins may also be increased depending on the age and gender of the victims, and also by the presence of comorbidities (e.g. pre-existing liver or gastrointestinal disease) [40]. Children are more susceptible to toxins because of their lower body weight, behavior, and toxic effects on development [41].

Adda ((2S, 3S, 8S, 9S) 3-amino-9-methoxy-2, 6, 8-trimethyl-10-phenyl-deca-4, 6-dienoic acid), a common bioactive compound derived from MCs congeners and NOD, imparts cytotoxins with toxicity (**Figure 2**) [42]. The highest concentration of cyanotoxins is usually contained within the cells (intracellular toxins), and a small amount, rarely above a few μg/L, is dissolved in the water (extracellular toxins) [3, 33]. Anatoxin-a and microcystin are mostly found intracellularly during the growth stage of the bloom. However, in cylindrospermopsin, the reported toxin ratio is about 50% intracellular and 50% extracellular. Extracellular toxins are more difficult to remove than intracellular toxins during drinking water purification, as they can absorb clays and organic material in the water column. The concentration of cyanotoxins significantly increases as a defense mechanism in stressful conditions (lack of nutrients/light) [43], also the death of cyanobacterial cells, at the end of their lifecycle or through measures taken during the control blooms, results in higher concentrations of extracellular toxin. The toxins in the cyanobacterial cells are still active for 21 days after the cell decays [44]. And most importantly, some cyanobacterial species show neurotoxic, hepatotoxic, and cytotoxic action despite not producing any known cyanotoxins [45–47]. These findings suggest the presence of potentially unknown or uncharacterized toxins, highlighting the necessity to explore and characterize potential new cyanobacterial toxins.

2.2 Exposure routes

Exposure to cyanotoxins can occur through a few main routes, which will be discussed roughly. Ingestion of contaminated water is one of the main routes of exposure and may occur through drinking water containing toxins or eating contaminated fish, shellfish, and bivalves. Irrigation of crops and plants with water contaminated with cyanotoxins is another way of possible intoxication. Bioaccumulation of cyanotoxins, and afterward, their bioavailability in the food chain is another prominent way of exposure that should be monitored more frequently (**Figure 3**). When cyanotoxins are released into the water, they can be ingested by aquatic invertebrates and aquatic vertebrates [48–50], and they have been found in plants [51], which poses a potential health risk to animals and humans through the food chain [52, 53]. Ingestion of some toxic amount of cyanotoxins may occur by consumption of nutritional supplements that contain blue-green algae as main or additional ingredients. Blue-green algae have a long history as a superfood for health (supports healthy digestion and strengthens the immune system, as a detoxifying agent, excellent fat burner, for

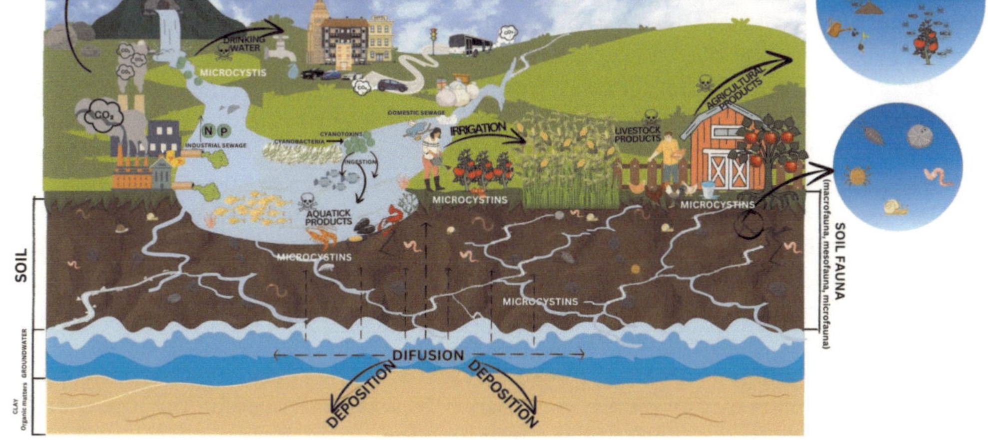

Figure 3.
Cyanotoxin incorporation through environment, jeopardizing human health and environment (Created by Author using Canva).

radioactive protection), skin's ultimate superfood (for eternal youth, skin pigmentation, moisturized skin, and improved skin structure), or medicine by humans for centuries [54]. Cyanobacteria are teeming with a high, unexhausted concentration of proteins, vitamins, minerals, carotenoids, and antioxidants which can promote optimal health in humans. In the United States, 38% of adults opted for alternative medicine over conventional drugs among patients with cardiovascular disease [55]. There has been an increasing demand for nutritional supplements for the prevention of COVID (SARS-CO2019). Mostly used are *Spirulina*, *Chlorella,* and *Aphanizomenon flos-aquae*, and some of them contain some groups of cyanotoxins at levels exceeding the tolerable daily intake values [56]. *Aph. flos-aquae* originated from the Upper Klamath Lake, Oregon, contaminated with high levels of MCs (up to 60 times higher than safety standards set by Oregon state) [57]. ATX-a and its congeners have been reported in different brands containing both *Spirulina* and *Aph. flos-aquae* [58, 59], and STX and BMAA in some strains of *Aph. flos-aquae* that are used for dietary supplements [60–62]. And more recently, the global war with COVID-19 raises a question—Could cyanobacterial metabolites be an immune booster against the COVID-19 pandemic, cause toxicosis, or even worse, worsen the condition of already developed lung diseases in patients with COVID? Boosting immunity has been a simple way to resist viral infection and limit fatalities [63, 64]. Cyanotoxins in supplements are a serious health risk. Nevertheless, the chemical composition, bioavailability, biological potency, toxicity, and related mechanisms of dietary supplements, respirators, and nasal sprays need to be investigated in detail [65].

Another prominent route of exposure to cyanotoxin is direct contact with the skin, through recreational activities, or beauty products based on cyanobacteria. During recreational activities on or near water bodies contaminated with cyanotoxins, a possible route of exposure is inhalation of aerosolized toxins. In recent years, an increased number of investigations have been recorded regarding the impact of aerosolized toxins [66–70]. In a conducted study [66], cyanobacteria were found at high frequencies in the upper respiratory tract (92.20%) and central airway (79.31%) with no relation to the specific time of year. The increasing spread of cyanobacterial blooms due to climate change and eutrophication worldwide may lead to an increase in aerosolized toxins and negative health effects. The growing populations and tourism near water bodies will further raise the number of people at risk. A population could be at risk for acute and chronic exposures as aerosolized cyanotoxins have been detected a few dozen kilometers away from the source [68]. The levels of aerosolized MCs fluctuated even when the concentrations in the water remained relatively stable. This highlights the significance of meteorological conditions (such as wind speed and direction) and aerosol generation mechanisms (such as wave breaking, spillway, and aeration systems) when assessing the risk of inhaling MCs and their potential impact on human health [70]. The potential chronic effects of cyanotoxins, particularly on vulnerable populations (with earlier noticed liver, gastrointestinal, or lung disease), require attention due to limited available data in this area. Understanding chronic, low-dose exposure to cyanotoxins is needed so that appropriate preventative, diagnostic, and therapeutic strategies can be created [40]. Widespread exposure to cyanobacterial toxins during bloom events in 2018 was evidenced by the presence of MCs in the nasal passages of 95% of the individuals previously studied in South Florida [71].

There are also documented cases of toxicosis by the intravenous route, through dialysis [72] where water sources from the clinique contained MCs and CYN.

2.3 Stability

Cyanotoxins are water-soluble and most of them are very stable in natural conditions due to their unreachable core structure. The cyanotoxins such as microcystin-LR (MC-LR) and STXs are persistent in the aquatic system and thus can directly enter the drinking water treatment. In addition, the half-life of MC-LR is around 90 days, and similarly, the half-life of STXs is approximately 9–28 days, which signifies their stability in natural water resources [73, 74]. MCs are extremely stable in water and only slowly decompose in acidic ($pH < 1$) and alkaline ($pH > 9$) conditions, exposed to high temperature (40°C), or by boiling [75], chemical, or biological degradation [76–79]. However, in most cases, bacteria able to degrade them are not present in the water, and therefore, toxins persist for months/years [78]. Their stability is provided by the cyclic structure and presence of novel amino acids. The cyclic structure of nodularins enables high chemical stability, which provides them resistance to boiling, chemical hydrolysis, and oxidation [80, 81]. Data show that nodularins degraded in negligible amounts while contained within living organisms [76, 77]. Cylindrospermopsin is stable at extreme temperatures, light, and pH, but is almost fully degraded when exposed to sunlight for 3 days [43]. ATX-a is unstable under natural conditions being partially or totally degraded and converted to non-toxic products (dihydroanatoxin-a and epoxyanatoxin-a) [82–84]. Anatoxin-a(S) is more soluble in water, which increases the rate of biodegradability compared to anatoxin-a. ATX-a(S) is unstable and inactivated at high temperatures (>40°C) or alkaline conditions [85]. Saxitoxins are water-soluble and stable toxins with persistence for more than 90 days in freshwater ecosystems [86]. In most cases, these compounds are progressively degraded into more toxic variants and in such conditions, may potentially increase toxicity. These facts, in combination with their high stability, represent a great problem for water treatment facilities and the implementation of an appropriate drinking water treatment.

3. Guideline values for cyanotoxins

As previously mentioned, cyanotoxin contamination of water bodies used for drinking or recreational purposes has become common. Reports of cyanotoxins poisoning incidents increase worldwide [2, 14], hence becoming health hazards globally [87]. The lack of official guidelines for cyanotoxin levels in drinking water has a great influence on risks to humans who use surface water which may be unsafe.

The risk of being exposed to toxic cyanobacteria and their toxins is high and will gradually be higher considering climate change and industrialization. Even with that emerging concern, a plan for the prevention of cyanobacterial blooming and regulations are still limited, even absent, in several countries. There are many different approaches dealing with the appearance of cyanobacterial blooms and cyanotoxins in freshwaters and drinking water reservoirs [36]. A number of countries (Canada, Brazil, New Zealand, and Australia) have developed regulations or guidelines for cyanotoxins and cyanobacteria in drinking water, and in some cases, in water used for recreational activity and agriculture (**Table 1**). In Kenya, there is a scarcity of information on cyanotoxins levels in domestic water sources, in Europe and the USA, and in several Latin American countries, there are no guidelines for any cyanotoxins in domestic water [88]. Despite the fact that there is no official federal legislation for cyanobacterial toxins in water with drinking purposes, Serbia has been working for almost 15 years on the analysis of the state of health and making precautionary measures, with special emphasis on the organization of the system for adequate information and health care [89]. Moreover, neighboring countries are affected by the same problem [34]. Argentina, Brazil, and Uruguay have conducted comprehensive studies to evaluate the distribution

Guideline values			**Reference**	**Guideline values**			**Reference**
Drinking water				**Recreational waters**			
MC	0.1 μg/L	Europe	[34, 94–102]	Relatively low risk**	2–4.0 μg/L MCs	20.000 cells/ml	[94]
	1.0 μg/L	Brazil (Regulatory Level); New Zealand; WHO*		Moderate significant risk***	>20.0 μg/L MCs	100.000 cells/ml	
	1.3 μg/L	Australia (Lifetime exposure); Canada		Situation of high risk****	>100.0 μg/L MCs	Appearance of visible aggregates	
	10.0 μg/L	Australia (Brief period)	[97, 102]				
NOD	1.0 μg/L	New Zealand	[95, 100, 103]	ND			
STX	0.1 μg/L	Europe	[96–98, 101–103]	ND			
	3.0 μg/L	Brazil (suggested); Australia (suggested); New Zealand					
ATX-a	0.1 μg/L	Europe	[96, 97, 100–102, 104–106]	ND			
	1.0 μg/L	According to Fawell					
	1.3 μg/L	Australia					
	1.5 μg/L	Canada					
	3.0 μg/L	Australia (suggested)					
	6.0 μg/L	New Zealand					
ATX-a(S)	1.0 μg/L	New Zealand	[100, 107]	ND			
HATX-a	2.0 μg/L	New Zealand	[100, 103]	ND			
CYN	0.1 μg/L	Europe	[96, 98, 101, 103]	ND			
	1.0 μg/L	New Zealand					
	1.0-15 μg/L	Australia					
	15.0 μg/L	Brazil (suggested)					
Dietary supplements							
1 ppm microcystins (ODA)			[94]				
Tolerable daily intake							
0.04 μg/kg/day			[94]				

**Brazil [98], China, Czech Republic, Finland, France [99], Japan, Italy, Denmark, Germany, Great Britain, Greece, Korea, New Zealand [101], Norway, Oregon (USA) [108], Poland, South Africa, Spain, USA [109]. **Czech Republic, France, Italy, Hungary, Turkey. ***Canada, Cuba, Czech Republic, France, Italy, Hungary, Turkey. ****France, Italy, Turkey.*

Table 1.
Guideline values for cyanotoxins.

of cyanobacterial blooms [90, 91], on the contrary for Peru, Chile, Colombia, and Venezuela, the information is limited to specific water bodies [92, 93].

Due to a lack of toxicity data for other toxins, in the reference [94], a provisional guideline for MC-LR has been set (1.0 μg/L for drinking water), hence cyanotoxins are not federally regulated contaminants. As a result, public drinking water providers are not required to routinely monitor drinking water for cyanotoxins. Setting up guideline values for cyanotoxins in drinking and recreational water and also in dietary supplements and cosmetics products is extremely crucial, so with that aim, **Table 1** presents legislation from different countries.

A provisional guideline value of 1 μg/L MC-LR in drinking water for human lifetime exposure and 12 μg/L for short-term exposure, respectively, was recommended by the World Health Organization (WHO) and value for CYN for human lifetime exposure is 0.7 μg/L [36]. Most of legislation are based on the WHO provisional value for drinking water, while others formulated their values, based upon local requirements (e.g. Czech Republic, France, Singapore, Uruguay, South Africa, Australia, Canada, New Zealand, South Korea, and Brazil) [35, 100]. Most countries define cyanotoxin concentration limits in drinking water but not in water used for recreational activities. The guideline value for the maximal acceptable concentration of MC-LR in drinking water was used also for human health risk assessment of microcystins resulting from recreational exposure, consumption of contaminated food, or food supplements [94, 110]. Brazil was the first country to enforce a specific, most comprehensive federal legislation for the control of cyanobacteria and their toxins in water used for drinking supply and recreational activities [100, 111, 112], which includes mandatory standard values for MCs, STXs, and CYN [113]. Concerning cyanotoxins, several countries have implemented monitoring programs based on cyanobacterial biomass for recreational water (cell numbers, chlorophyll-a concentration, and often cyanotoxin concentration) [94].

Due to the lack of relevant guideline values for other types of toxins, they might exhibit greater health risks to humans. Also, there might be a high level of unregulated cyanotoxin congeners, thereby posing unknown health risks. The definition of guideline values for all types of cyanotoxins is needed as the current regulations are insufficient, especially in developing countries and rural areas. Despite the risks associated with cyanotoxins, current regulations for dietary supplements are insufficient to safeguard consumers. These guidelines should determine the values of cyanotoxins in accordance with patients with chronic illnesses and kids. Kids are more susceptible than school-age children through adults considering they consume more water relative to their body weight [14].

4. Drinking water supply: occurrence of cyanobacteria and water treatment for cyanotoxin removal

4.1 Cyanobacteria and cyanotoxins in drinking water supply

Based on previous literature data, it is clear that almost every part of the world has or will encounter problems with toxic cyanobacteria in its drinking water system. The occurrence of toxic cyanobacterial blooms is increasing in frequency and distribution [2], and so does the chance of losing access to safe drinking water. Of all the routes of cyanotoxin exposure to humans, drinking water is the main source. Despite having a sufficient quantity of water, availability may be limited if the quality does not meet the requirements for its intended use. The increased occurrence of toxic cyanobacteria and cyanotoxins is increasingly being viewed as a contaminant of emerging concern and is considered a major health risk related to surface waters worldwide, which further increases the cost of water resources. This problem was cumulated in Lake Vrutci (Užice, Serbia), where the presence of cyanobacteria *Planktothrix rubescens* was documented, with the presence of MC-LR in the fish tissue, lake, and the tap water, as well as other types of MCs detected [114]. During this period, 70,000 people living in Užice were left without healthy drinking water. Because of contaminated water with the bloom of *Microcystis* sp. in Toledo, Ohio, a public advisory shutdown the water supply for 3 days which impacted over 400,000 people [115]. In 2013, in finished drinking water of Carroll Township, Ohio was detected at 1.4 mg/L and 3.6 mg/L of MCs equivalents, and water has been out of use for the 2200 population. Another well-known drinking water crisis has affected municipalities on the shores of Lake Taihu (China), Lake Erie (Ohio, USA) [6], and in July 2018, Greenfield, Iowa; in 2007, residents from Changchun and two million people from Wuxi (Jiangsu Province) went without drinking water due to a cyanobacterial bloom occurrence. The current circumstances compel millions of people to purchase bottled drinking water. Continuous exposure to cyanotoxins in drinking water may reach a lethal dose within the human lifespan, leading to death, in some cases, or in negligible levels, can cause carcinogenicity [114, 116]. Safe drinking water remains a challenge worldwide in many rural communities [36], which causes 1.2 million deaths per year [117, 118].

Mass occurrences of toxic cyanobacteria and their toxins in reservoirs represent a great challenge for the production of safe drinking water through the application of adequate water treatment techniques.

4.2 Water treatment for cyanotoxin removal from drinking water supply

Drinking water sources pose a great challenge for drinking water facilities. Fresh cyanobacterial blooms often smell like fresh-cut grass, while older blooms can stink like pig pens. Older blooms are more likely to release toxins when dying as their cells break down. Filamentous cyanobacteria cause problems in water treatment systems by clogging in filters for drinking water supply. In that manner, during the water treatment process, cyanobacterial cells, odor, and color need to be reduced and cyanotoxins eliminated. The mass presence of the potentially toxic cyanobacteria represents a real threat to human and animal health, and an important indicator of the rapid water quality deterioration [119], which further poses a serious problem to water treatment facilities because not all water treatment technologies can remove all cyanotoxins below acceptable levels [4]. The health issues caused by cyanotoxins presence have led to efforts by water suppliers to develop effective treatments and management approaches for the production of safe drinking water. To minimize the risk from cyanotoxins in drinking water, a multi-barrier approach is needed; incorporating prevention, source control, adequate treatment, and a monitoring system. Prevention of bloom appearance is a crucial step as a defense mechanism over invasive cyanobacterial blooms in water reservoirs. Bad management of water purification systems can lead to serious problems.

A lot of cases are documented where the treatment process previously used was ineffective against cyanobacterial blooms which caused serious human poisoning likewise 2000 cases of gastroenteritis and diarrhea, including 88 deaths after drinking boiled water from the dam [120]; gastrointestinal illness among 9000 people receiving drinking water from rivers in West Virginia [121]; gastroenteritis with abdominal pain and vomiting affecting 5000–8000 persons where drinking water treatment by precipitation, filtration, and chlorination was not sufficient to remove the toxins in Ohio river [122, 123]; or gastroenteritis with vomiting and headache among 149 persons in Australia, Solomon Dam, where treating bloom with copper sulfate resulted in the liberation of toxins [124]. Serious human poisonings happened in Charleston, West Virginia even precipitation, filtration, and chlorination were applied [125]. Drinking water supply without a proper basic drinking water purification process in Zimbabwe, Africa, caused gastroenteritis, skin rashes, itching, and eye sores in children [126]. Also, there is animal intoxication cases after drinking contaminated water, for example, several hundred livestock died within hours in Australia [127, 128], in South Africa [129], Switzerland [130], Sweden [131], and the USA [132–135]. When inappropriate treatment was used, cyanobacteria cells were not degraded, stayed intact after water treatment, and caused blooms in the post-treatment drinking water tanks. In reservoir Vrutci, Serbia slow-sand filtration was applied, but was not a sufficient method that led to sickness of people and deaths of animals [114], also people who use water from Malpas Dam, Armidale experienced serious chronic effects like liver damage [136, 137], or in China development of primary liver cancer [138, 139].

Most cyanotoxins are cell-bound and are released when the cells age, die, or are lysed through employed purification systems [140, 141], which present a hazard to animals and humans using the water, especially when used as a potable water source. Not all countries have appropriate means to deal with cyanobacteria problems, as well as sensitive and precise analytical methods for cyanotoxin detection, which are usually expensive and inaccessible. However, over 300 analogs of MCs have been identified, but not all are presently monitored, therefore, any conclusions based only on the presence of MC-LR can be misleading. Chronic exposure to low concentrations of MC increases the risk of developing cancer (e.g. China, Florida, Serbia). This situation can be linked to the country where the populations receive drinking water from surface accumulations that are frequently blooming [142]. The unequal geographical distribution of liver cancer in Serbia was visible and outbreaks can be correlated with drinking water supplies, where districts with a higher risk of developing primary liver cancer are using reservoirs that are continuously blooming, and low-risk regions have purification systems of drinking water [142].

Different techniques have to be included in order to reduce cyanobacterial growth and cyanotoxins [3]. Effective removal of cyanobacterial toxins depends on the type and concentrations of chemicals used in the water treatment processes, also physical parameters of water (e.g. pH and the contact time), as well as concentrations and types of cyanotoxins entering the treatment and also varies among cyanobacterial species (**Table 2**). For example, chloramine is the least effective oxidant for inactivating *Microcystis aeruginosa*, *Oscillatoria* sp., and *Lyngbya* sp. [143], and coagulation/flocculation/sedimentation completely removes cells of, for example, *Aphanizomenon flos-aquae*, *Merismopedia* sp., *Phormidium corium*, while *M. aeruginosa* and *Gloeocapsa* sp. were intact [144]. MCs have been reported in final drinking water in many countries including Argentina, Australia, Bangladesh, Canada, Czech Republic, China, Finland, France, Germany, Latvia, Poland, Thailand, Turkey, Serbia, Spain, Switzerland, and the USA [121, 122]. A survey of 45 drinking water supplies in Canada and the United States detected MC in 80% of the raw and treated water observed, but only 4% of the samples exceeded the WHO drinking water guideline [145].

From all the statements from **Table 2**, it could be concluded that no single treatment method can remove all contaminants from water, thus more efficient and cost-effective technology needs to be developed. Water treatment can be highly effective

Treatment technique		**Expected removal**		**Additional comments**
		Intracellular	**Extracellular**	
Auxiliary process				
Pre-ozonation		Auxiliary process	—	Auxiliary process for enhancing coagulation, however this process can lead to toxin release.
Pre-chlorination	Pre-chlorination	Auxiliary process	—	Useful to assist coagulation of cells, with subsequent treatment steps which will remove dissolved toxins. Depends on the type of chlorine.
	Free chlorine	—	> 100%	Effective on degradation of microcystin, cylindrospermopsin, and saxitoxin, but not for anatoxin-a.
	Chloramine	—	Negligible	Ineffective.
	Chlorine dioxide	—	Negligible	Ineffective (with doses used in drinking water treatment).
Conventional water treatment				
Coagulation	Coagulation	> 90%	< 10%	This treatment may cause lysis of cyanobacterial cells. NOM decrease removal efficiencies.
	Ferrate oxidation-coagulation	—	> 93%	This process has advantage over using chlorine, ozone or peroxide for oxidation.
Filtration	Slow sand filtration	<86%	Probably significant	Very useful if combinated with other water treatments.
	Rapid filtration	>60%	<10%	This method causes lysis of cyanobacterial cells. Usually employed after coagulation to remove the particles.
	Membrane processes	>96%	Uncertain	Effective in the removal of whole cells. Depends on pore size of RO and NF membranes, and water quality, dissolved MCs have been removed. This treatment causes cells lysis.
Absorption	PAC	Negligible	>85%	Effective in toxin removal but with very high doses of PAC. Generally effective for removal of MC, ATX-a and CYN. DOC will reduce capacity. It has to change frequently which significantly increased treatment costs.
	GAC	>60%	>95%	DOC competition and presence of NOM decreases toxin adsorption process. GAC filters with proper replacement can be used as an auxiliary barrier for MC, but less effective for ATX-a and CYN.
	Biological GAC	Excellent	>90%	Better effectiveness in toxin removal than GAC.
Ozonation	Potassium permanganate	—	95%	Advantages: low cost, ease of handling, effectiveness over a wide pH range; Disadvantages: long contact time, gives water pink color, toxic, cause skin irritation, fatal if swallowed.
	Ozonation	—	>98%	It is best to use oxidation to degrade dissolved cyanotoxins after the removal of algal cells by

Treatment technique		Expected removal		Additional comments
		Intracellular	**Extracellular**	
				a coagulation and filtration. The initial cost of ozonation equipment is high, ozone is highly corrosive and toxic, and requires higher level of maintenance and operator skill; leads to cell lysis.
	Hydrogen peroxide	—	Uncertain	Not effective on its own.
Advanced oxidation technologies (AOTs)				
AOTs	UV radiation/ AOTs	—	Negligible	Effective in removing of MC-LR, ATX-a, and CYN, but only at impractically high doses. Because of the high doses required, low to medium pressure lamp, UV treatment is not recommended as a viable treatment barrier for cyanotoxins. Leads to lysis of the cell wall.
	Titanium dioxide/AOTs	—	100%	One of the most promising AOTs, inexpensive and photocatalytic active catalyst under UV and visible light; without utilizing or producing hazardous compounds. This treatment resulted in complete degradation of the cyanotoxin under UV light.
	Fenton and Photo-Fenton processes	—	60–100%	Fenton process depends on the pH, concentration of H_2O_2 and Fenton reagent. The highest degradation efficiency was achieved when UV radiation was involved, during the Photo-Fenton process.
	Sonolysis	—	Reduction of algae cells	Best if applied with AOTs. Significantly enhance reduction of algae cells, without lysis of cells. Application of ultrasonic irradiation requires frequencies that lead to extreme conditions. Without chemical addition.
	Biodegradation	—	100%	*Sphingomonas* sp., *Paucibacter toxinivorans gen. Nov. Sp. nov*, *Burkholderia*, *Arthrobacter* sp., *Brevibacterium* sp., *Rhodococcus* sp., and *Methylobacillus* sp. are capable to degrading some types of cyanotoxins. Better in conjunction with UV/H_2O_2, ozone, PAC, or GAC. Advantages: reliable, cost-effective, which does not involve any use of harmful chemicals; disadvantages: long reaction time of hours to days.

Abbreviations: AOTs-advanced oxidation technologies; ATX-anatoxins; ATX-a(S)-antoxin-a (S); CYN-cylindrospermopsin; DOC-dissolved organic carbon; GAC-granular activated carbon; MC-microcystins; NF-nanofiltrattion; NOD-nodularin; NOM-natural organic matter; PAC-powdered activated carbon; RO-reverse osmosis; STX-saxitoxins.

Table 2.
Effectiveness of water treatment on removal of cyanotoxins.

in removing cyanobacterial cells and toxins (especially MCs) with the appropriate combination of treatments. Some most common treatments of water contaminated with cyanobacterial blooms use pre-oxidants (such as ozone, chlorine, chlorine dioxide, chloramine, potassium permanganate, ferrate, and copper sulfate) which while killing cells will result in the release of cyanotoxins [146], so demand subsequent step to remove dissolved extracellular toxins (**Table 2**). Further processes involve conventional water treatment-coagulation, flocculation, and absorption (sedimentation). Coagulation provides high removal rates of intracellular toxins (> 90%), and somewhat less important of extracellular toxins (< 10%), but this process may cause lysis of cyanobacterial cells. Coagulation supplemented with ferrate (ferrate oxidation-coagulation) has an advantage over using chlorine, ozone, or peroxide for oxidation, with expected removal rates of less than 93% for extracellular toxins, and negligible for intracellular toxins. Filtration is very useful if combined with other water treatments, and usually is employed after coagulation to remove the particles. Slow sand filtration provides the removal of intracellular toxins over 86%, and rapid filtration less than 60%. Membrane filtration processes are effective in the removal of whole cells, depending on the pore size of RO and NF membranes, and water quality. However, filtration causes cell lysis and promotes the increase of dissolved cyanotoxins [4, 146]. The removal efficiency of cyanobacterial cells with conventional water processes is species-specific [144], however, the established opinion is that these treatments were insufficient for the complete removal of cyanobacterial cells, especially of toxins [144, 147]. Given the lack of cyanotoxin removal using coagulation and filtration, a possible way to eliminate cyanotoxins below the WHO guidelines value is the application of these treatments combined with the addition of PAC/GAC. PAC is effective for the removal of MC, ATX-a, and CYN, and GAC for MC, but less effective for ATX-a and CYN [4]. Absorption has excellent removal of extracellular toxins, with PAC less than 85%, and GAC 95%. The choice of a form of activated carbon (PAC or GAC) is typically a function of operating conditions. When using GAC, the formation of biofilms (biological GAC) can occur which has been shown to give higher cyanotoxin removal [148]. A further step for improvement of the water purification system is ozonation, which degrades dissolved cyanotoxins after the removal of algal cells by coagulation, filtration, and sedimentation. Usage of ozonation achieves removal of extracellular toxins higher than 98%. However, the equipment required for ozonization is demanding, keeping in mind that ozone is highly corrosive and toxic, and requires a higher level of maintenance and operator skill; also leads to cell lysis. The application of hydrogen peroxide has shown uncertain toxin removal. Potassium permanganate accomplishes the removal of extracellular toxins up to 95%, and as an advantage, it is inexpensive, easy to handle, and effective over a wide pH range. However, this treatment is toxic and can cause skin irritation, and it can be fatal if swallowed. Advanced oxidation processes (AOTs) involve the use of UV, UV/H_2O_2, ultrasound, and ozone. The most recent study [149] showed that the removal rate of *M. aeruginosa* increased with the extension of time and the removal effect of static ultrasound was better than with dynamic ultrasound. However, the release of toxins was less in dynamic ultrasound radiation. UV radiation/AOTs is effective in removing MC-LR, ATX-a, and CYN, but only at impractically high doses, therefore is not recommended as a step in treatments for cyanotoxins. Titanium dioxide/AOTs is one of the most promising AOTs (expected removal: intracellular toxins negligible, extracellular 100%), inexpensive, and photocatalytic active catalyst under UV and visible light, without utilizing or producing hazardous compounds. This treatment completes degraded cyanotoxins under UV light. The Fenton process (for intracellular toxins - ineffective, for extracellular - 60–100% effectiveness) depends on the pH, concentration of H_2O_2, and Fenton reagent. The highest degradation efficiency was achieved when UV radiation was involved, during the Photo-Fenton process. Sonolysis is best if applied with AOTs, significantly enhances the reduction of algae cells without lysis of cells. The application of ultrasonic irradiation requires frequencies that lead to extreme conditions. Biodegradation is being explored as a treatment for the efficient removal of cyanotoxins from drinking water, with the expected removal of extracellular toxins of 100%. *Sphingomonas* sp. [150, 151], *Paucibacter toxinivorans* gen. Nov. Sp. nov, *Burkholderia*, *Arthrobacter* sp., *Brevibacterium* sp., *Rhodococcus* sp., and *Methylobacillus* sp. [152, 153] are capable of degrading some types of cyanotoxins. Biological degradation is better in conjunction with UV/H_2O_2, ozone, PAC, or GAC. This treatment is reliable, cost-effective, does not involve the use of harmful chemicals, and has a long reaction time of hours to days. Advanced oxidation processes show promising results for the destruction of intact cyanobacterial cells and cyanotoxins in drinking water.

MCs, ATX-a, CYN, and some STXs are adsorbed from the solution by both granular activated carbon and, less efficiently, by powdered activated carbon. Adequate contact time and pH are needed to achieve optimal removal of cyanotoxins. Therefore, the practice of prechlorination or pre-ozonation is not recommended without a subsequent step to remove dissolved cyanobacterial toxins. So, **Figure 4** provides our model for a sufficient purification system of water contaminated with cyanobacteria.

The problem regarding cyanobacteria and their toxins in water bodies is an urgent matter and should be changed in the near future. The monitoring of water supply systems for cyanobacteria and cyanotoxins, especially reservoirs for drinking purposes, is not yet common practice in most of the countries in the world. Therefore,

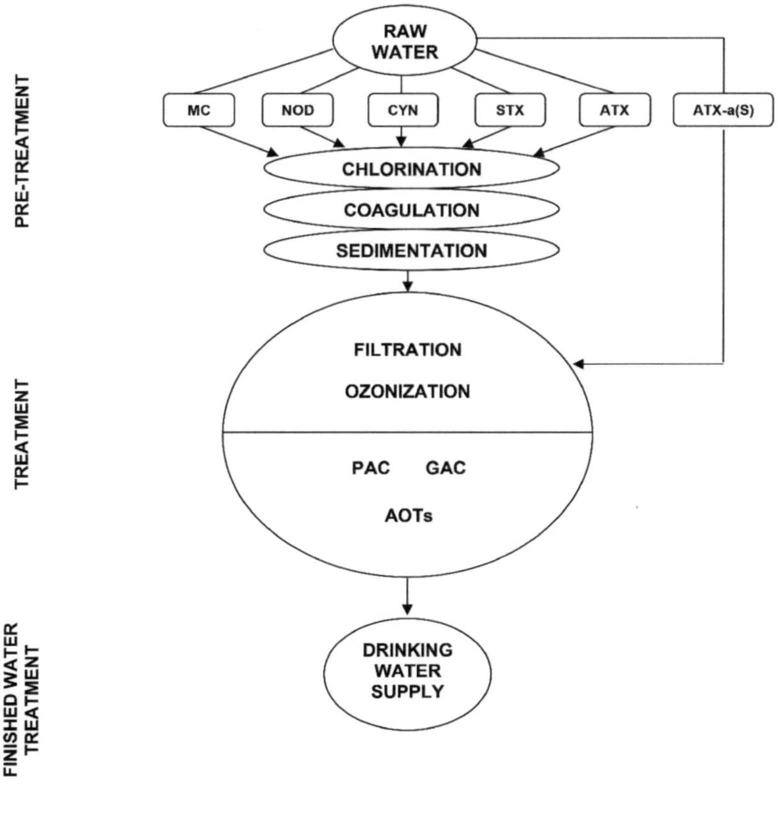

Figure 4.
Water treatments specific to certain cyanotoxins. Abbreviations: AOTs-advanced oxidation technologies; ATX-anatoxins; ATX-a(S)-antoxin-a (S); CYN-cylindrospermopsin; GAC-granular activated carbon; MC-microcystins; NOD-nodularin; PAC-powdered activated carbon; STX-saxitoxins.

various techniques and methods in water treatment procedures must be employed as necessary measures for the preservation of the local environment, and water quality. Furthermore, financial support plays an important obstacle, when it comes to cyanotoxin monitoring and treatment measurements implementation. All points which are given in previous paragraphs point out the harmfulness of cyanobacteria and their toxins and implicate the necessity of introduction of legislation concerning the determination and monitoring of these toxins. To avoid risks to human health, an appropriate drinking water treatment is necessary for cyanotoxin elimination from water, which poses a great problem, as some treatment leads to cell lysis and the release of cyanotoxins, which are mostly water-soluble. **Table 2** (supplemented with **Figure 4**) addresses the methods available for its removal and also the difficulties faced in each process. Treatments that have been proven to reduce cyanotoxins below toxic levels include activated carbon, slow sand filtration, conventional filtration, membrane filtration, advanced UV, and ozone [4]. Assessment of water treatment procedures has shown that most methods would result in a reduction of cyanobacterial toxins concentrations below the WHO guideline value of 1 μg/L drinking water [108]. It is important to emphasize that most of the water treatments are developed for successful MC-LR elimination, as it is the most common toxin found in aquatic environments. However, these treatments do not guarantee the successful elimination of other known MC equivalents (>300) and other groups of cyanotoxins that can occur. Therefore, the development of various robust, accurate, and affordable techniques and methods in water treatment procedures must be employed as necessary measures for the preservation of the local environment and water quality. Although satellite remote sensing technology cannot detect cyanotoxins [154], they can be used for detecting and quantifying cyanobacterial bloom abundance [155]. This method can help prioritize locations with greater exposure to blooms and is used to assist in prioritizing management actions for water with drinking and recreational purposes and may provide an indicator for human and ecological health protection (hypoxic events, phytoplankton composition, light availability) [156–158]. A few recent studies have shown that the detection and quantification of cyanotoxins (MCs) in water can be achieved with passive samplers, which can be used effectively at low levels (of μg/L and ng/L) of toxins [159–162]. The study [161] monitored MC levels in different stages of water treatment, and also at different depths of the lake. Nowadays, there are different commercially available passive samplers, like polar organic compound integrative sampler (POCIS), Chemcatcher (passive water quality sampler for micropollutants), or SPATT devices (specialized for cyanotoxins).

5. Proposed therapy for cyanobacterial blooms intoxications

Toxicoses caused by cyanotoxins are a serious condition that requires immediate medical attention to prevent fatality. Based on available literature, diagnostic tests for cyanotoxins are currently not available for clinical use. The fact that robust, inexpensive, and widely accessible assays are not available to facilitate rapid diagnosis and therapy of cyanobacterial intoxication represents a crucial problem in the modern health system. As previously mentioned, the significant number of poisoning cases caused by cyanotoxins, and the potential for future increases in such cases, underscores the urgent need to develop effective therapies. These therapies should eventually be incorporated into standard treatment practices. The detection of cyanotoxins in blood, respiratory mucosa, and urine samples to diagnose acute or chronic intoxication is difficult and requires sophisticated, expansive analysis techniques. Some specialized laboratories can perform tests (electrolytes and liver enzymes; renal function tests, serum glucose, and urine tests; chest radiographs) to identify intoxications caused by the presence of cyanobacteria/cyanotoxins.

It is important to find simple and quick methods to address this issue. As the occurrence of toxic cyanobacterial blooms and human exposures become more common, the recently developed method [163] using Immunocapture-Protein Phosphatase Inhibition Assay may be used as a simple and robust assay to detect cyanotoxins (MCs) in human plasma. Unlike previous methods that engage in acute exposure to MCs [164–167], this method was developed for the detection of low-level MC exposures (through inhalation) [163]. Studies performed earlier have detected MCs in urine samples (mouse and human), plasma (mouse), and serum samples (mouse and human) [164–167]. Previously, quantification of MC and NOD concentration was measured in human urine by Immunocapture-Protein Phosphatase Inhibition assay [165]; MCs by a simple colorimetric method [167], or in urine, plasma, and serum through development and applications of solid-phase extraction and liquid chromatography-mass spectrometry methods [166]. The presence of specific antibodies in serum could be used as exposure biomarkers to complement epidemiological studies and medical diagnosis of cyanotoxin intoxications.

There are no antidotes for cyanotoxins [168]. Decontamination, administration of cholestyramine, and symptomatic therapy in combination with supportive care consisting of fluids, mucosal protectants, vitamins, antibiotics, and nutritional supplements may be considered as one of the strategies in cases of toxicities with cyanobacteria [169]. Respiratory support may provide sufficient time for detoxication followed by recovery of respiratory control [168]. Therefore, a crucial step in future studies is introducing adequate therapy in case of cyanotoxin poisonings for treating both animal and human cases.

6. Limitations

There are some limitations that will be a problem in future research regarding cyanotoxins in water bodies for drinking and recreational use. The primary limitation is that the number of cases analyzed in the literature is limited to available reports, databases, and literature published so far. The data are unavailable or limited in many countries (e.g. Argentina, Chile, Paraguay, Colombia) [170, 171]. Also, the number of scientists and interest in the field of health and environment are scarce in rural regions and developing countries [2]. Research on cyanotoxins and cyanobacteria, as well as the number of reported cases, varies among the countries, where financial support plays an important role. Also, insufficient medical and veterinary training and knowledge of the public community are recognized in developing countries and rural regions. There was a correlation between the level of education and the number of reported symptoms, with higher education levels associated with fewer reported symptoms [69]. Moreover, there is no routine monitoring of cyanotoxins in freshwater bodies. Laws and regulations in different countries mostly do not oblige monitoring of cyanotoxins, therefore, the actual number of cases is most likely higher than reported.

According to the latest data, there are over 300 different MC variants [31], and drinking water treatments and toxicity tests are usually tested only for MC-LR. Standards for cyanotoxins detection are very expensive, and unreachable; also there is demand for (expensive) equipment and highly educated technicians. So main question is: What about other groups of cyanotoxins? For some groups of cyanotoxins, there are no standards. They are all present in the water but unmonitored and pass by, undercovered. And just like that, silently, they change the environment and cause health issues. More recently published information of toxic effects caused by cyanobacterial species that cannot produce cyanotoxins increases the importance of preventing the appearance of cyanobacteria, and furthermore of their safe removal from water bodies intended for drinking and recreational purposes.

Thorough, detailed overcoming of limitations is the key to combating powerful cyanobacteria.

7. Conclusion

Available, bacteriologically safe drinking water is essential. The government aims to tackle the issue of water scarcity, particularly in rural areas, where residents are impoverished and unable to access clean, safe drinking water. An appropriate drinking water treatment is necessary to eliminate cyanobacteria and their toxins from the water. A combination of different, advanced treatments for cyanotoxin removal should be performed. However, their elimination from the drinking water supply is challenging. Different types of cyanotoxins, even metabolites from non-toxin-producing species, have different characteristics, stability, and structure. Depending on the source organisms, they can be distributed at different depths through water samples. Therefore, the most important thing in the fight against cyanobacteria is the spread of knowledge, the prevention of their appearance and spread, and appropriate behavior when they appear on the water surface.

Sharing knowledge about the environmental conditions that encourage bloom formation and their toxins is crucial for managing the risks associated with cyanobacterial toxin issues. The medical employees and also residents have to be capable of recognizing the occurrence of cyanobacterial blooms and how to behave accordingly. The deepest research is necessary to identify populations with underlying comorbidities that may increase susceptibility to cyanotoxin exposure and to develop an adequate therapy for treating animal and human cases caused by cyanotoxin intoxication. A crucial step in the improvement of the cyanotoxin control system is the setting guideline values for all cyanotoxins, which also includes monitoring their fate in aquatic food chains, during food processing, and routine control of food supplements and healthy food.

A future study should focus on determining potentially harmful cyanobacterial compounds, and all types of cyanotoxins in water reservoirs, and expand studies related to cyanotoxins in countries in development. A diagnostic test that does not require a standard for detection is necessary to identify toxicoses. The data gathered indicates the need for future research to focus on developing reliable and precise, yet affordable and widely accessible, analytical techniques for detecting cyanotoxins, available to wealthier and developing countries, and also to rural aeries. The incorporation of new methodologies, likewise passive samplers, satellite-based remote sensing tools, or *in vivo* pigment fluorescence, could provide consistent, low-cost data for the development of large geographical monitoring programs and should be considered for analysis carefully in future studies.

Acknowledgements

This work was supported by the Ministry of Science, Technological Development and Innovation of the Republic of Serbia (Grants No. 451-03-66/2024-03/200125 & 451-03-65/2024-03/200125).

I would like to express my deepest appreciation to my dear colleague Dr. Gorenka Bojadžija Savić for helpful contributions, constructive advice, and insightful suggestions.

Conflict of interest

The author declares no conflict of interest.

Abbreviations

AOTs	advanced oxidation technologies
ATX-a	anatoxin-a
ATX-a(S)	anatoxin-a(S)
BMAA	β-N-methylamino-L-alanine
CYN	cylindrospermopsin
GAC	granular activated carbon
LPS	lipopolysaccharides
MC	microcystin
MC-LR	microcystin-LR
NOD	nodularin
NOM	natural organic matter
NSTX	neosaxitoxin
PAC	powdered activated carbon
RO	reverse osmosis
STX	saxitoxin
WHO	World Health Organization

Author details

Dijana Lalić
Faculty of Sciences, Department of Biology and Ecology, University of Novi Sad, Serbia

*Address all correspondence to: dijana.pantelic@dbe.uns.ac.rs

References

[1] Lalić D, Meriluoto J, Zorić M, Dulić T, Mirosavljević M, Župunski M, et al. Potential of cyanobacterial secondary metabolites as biomarkers for paleoclimate reconstruction. Catena. 2020;**185**:104283

[2] Svirčev Z, Lalić D, Bojadžija Savić G, Tokodi N, Drobac Backović D, Chen L, et al. Global geographical and historical overview of cyanotoxin distribution and cyanobacterial poisonings. Archives of Toxicology. 2019;**93**:2429-2248

[3] Chorus I, Bartram J, editors. Toxic Cyanobacteria in Water: A Guide for their Public Health Consequences, Monitoring and Management. London, New York: Published on behalf of WHO by E&FN Spon; 1999

[4] Pantelić D, Svirčev Z, Simeunović J, Vidović M, Trajković I. Cyanotoxins: Characteristics, production and degradation routes in drinking water treatment with reference to the situation in Serbia. Chemosphere. 2013;**91**: 421-441

[5] Munoz M, Cirés S, de Pedro ZM, Colina JA, Velásquez-Figueroa Y, et al. Overview of toxic cyanobacteria and cyanotoxins in Ibero-American freshwaters: Challenges for risk management and opportunities for removal by advanced technologies. Science of the Total Environment. 2021; **761**:143197

[6] Huisman J, Codd GA, Paerl HW, Ibelings BW, Verspagen JM, Visser PM. Cyanobacterial blooms. Nature Reviews. Microbiology. 2018;**16**(8):471

[7] Kulabhusan PK, Campbell KV. Physico-chemical treatments for the removal of cyanotoxins from drinking water: Current challenges and future trends. Science of the Total Environment. 2024;**917**:170078

[8] Lopez CB, Jewett EB, Dortch Q, Walton BT, Hudnell HK. Scientific assessment of freshwater harmful algal blooms. Washington, DC: Interagency Working Group on Harmful Algal Blooms, Hypoxia, and Human Health of the Joint Subcommittee on Ocean Science and Technology; 2008

[9] Paerl HW, Huisman J. Climate change: A catalyst for global expansion of harmful cyanobacterial. Blooms. Environmental Microbiology Reports. 2009;**1**:27-37

[10] Neilan BA, Pearson LA, Muenchhoff J, Moffitt MC, Dittmann E. Environmental conditions that influence toxin biosynthesis in cyanobacteria. Environmental Microbiology. 2013;**15**: 1239-1253

[11] Schulhof MA, Shurin JB, Declerck SAJ, Van de Waal DB. Phytoplankton growth and stoichiometric responses to warming, nutrient addition and grazing depend on Lake productivity and cell size. Global Change Biology. 2019;**25**: 2751-2762

[12] Walls JT, Wyatt KH, Doll JC, Rubenstein EM, Rober AR. Hot and toxic: Temperature regulates microcystin release from cyanobacteria. Science of the Total Environment. 2018;**610**: 786-795

[13] Miller T, Beversdorf L, Weirich C, Bartlett S. Cyanobacterial toxins of the Laurentian Great Lakes, their toxicological effects, and numerical limits in drinking water. Marine Drugs. 2017;**15**(6):160

[14] EPA. Cyanobacteria and Cyanotoxins: Information for Drinking Water Systems. United States: United States Environmental Protection Agency Office of Water; 2019; EPA-810F11001

[15] Wurtsbaugh WA, Paerl HW, Dodds WK. Nutrients, eutrophication and harmful algal blooms along the freshwater to marine continuum. WIREs Water. 2019;**6**(5):e1373

[16] Downing TG, Sember CS, Gehringer MM, Leukes W. Medium N: P ratios and specific growth rate comodulate microcystin and protein content in *Microcystis aeruginosa* PCC7806 and *M. aeruginosa* UV027. Microbial Ecology. 2005;**49**:468-473

[17] Polyak Y, Zaytseva T, Medvedeva N. Response of toxic cyanobacterium *Microcystis aeruginosa* to environmental pollution. Water, Air, and Soil Pollution. 2013;**224**:1-14

[18] Martínez-Ruiz EB, Martínez-Jerónimo F. How do toxic metals affect harmful cyanobacteria? An integrative study with a toxigenic strain of *Microcystis aeruginosa* exposed to nickel stress. Ecotoxicology and Environmental Safety. 2016;**133**:36-46

[19] Doubek JP, Carey CC. Catchment, morphometric, and water quality characteristics differ between reservoirs and naturally formed lakes on a latitudinal gradient in the coterminous United States. Inland Waters. 2017;**7**:171-180

[20] Tee HS, Waite D, Payne L, Middleditch M, Wood S, Handley KM. Tools for successful proliferation: Diverse strategies of nutrient acquisition by a benthic cyanobacterium. The ISME Journal. 2020;**14**(8):2164-2178

[21] Ji F, Wu Z, Huang J, Chassignet EP. Evolution of land surface air temperature trend. Nature Climate Change. 2014;**4**:462-466

[22] Reynolds CS. Cyanobacterial water blooms. In: Callow JA, editor. Advances in Botanical Research. London: Academic Press; 1987. pp. 67-143

[23] Carpenter S, Brock W, Cole J, Kitchell J, Pace M. Leading indicators of trophic cascades. Ecology Letters. 2008;**11**(2):128-138

[24] Cao H, Han L, Li L. A deep learning method for cyanobacterial harmful algae blooms prediction in Taihu Lake, China. Harmful Algae. 2022;**113**:102189

[25] Bláha L, Babica P, Maršálek B. Toxins produced in cyanobacterial water bloom–toxicity and risks. Interdisciplinary Toxicology. 2009;**2**(2):36-41

[26] Jahn M, Vialas V, Karlsen J, Maddalo G, Edfors F, Forsström B, et al. Growth of cyanobacteria is constrained by the abundance of light and carbon assimilation proteins. Cell Reports. 2018;**25**(2):478-486.e8

[27] Kang BK, Park J. Effect of input variable characteristics on the performance of an ensemble machine learning model for algal bloom prediction. Journal of Korean Society of Water and Wastewater. 2021;**35**(6):417-424

[28] Yuan J, Cao Z, Ma J, Li Y, Qiu Y, Duan H. Influence of climate extremes on long-term changes in cyanobacterial blooms in a eutrophic and shallow lake. Science of the Total Environment. 2024;**939**:173601

[29] Hartnell DM, Chapman IJ, Taylor NGH, Esteban GF, Turner AD,

Franklin DJ. Cyanobacterial abundance and microcystin profiles in two southern British Lakes: The importance of abiotic and biotic interactions. Toxins. 2020; **12**(8):503

[30] Coffer MM, Schaeffer BA, Salls WB, Urquhart E, Loftin KA, Stumpf RP, et al. Satellite remote sensing to assess cyanobacterial bloom frequency across the United States at multiple spatial scales. Ecological Indicators. 2021;**128**: 107822

[31] Baliu-Rodriguez D, Peraino NJ, Premathilaka SH, Birbeck JA, Baliu-Rodriguez T, Westrick JA, et al. Identification of novel microcystins using high-resolution MS and MSn with python code. Environmental Science & Technology. 2022;**56**(3):1652-1663

[32] Yang Y, Yu G, Chen Y, Jia N, Li R. Four decades of progress in cylindrospermopsin research: The ins and outs of a potent cyanotoxin. Journal of Hazardous Materials. 2021;**406**: 124653

[33] Codd GA. The Toxicity of Benthic Blue-Green Algae in Scottish Freshwaters. Marlow, UK: Foundation for Water Research; 1995

[34] Codd GA, Morrison LF, Metcalf JS. Cyanobacterial toxins: Risk management for health protection. Toxicology and Applied Pharmacology. 2005;**203**: 264-272

[35] Sanseverino I, António DC, Loos R, Lettieri T. Cyanotoxins: Methods and Approaches for their Analysis and Detection. Europian Comission; JRC106478; EUR 28624 EN; 2017

[36] World Health Organization. Background Document for Development of WHO Guidelines for Drinking-Water Quality and Guidelines for Safe Recreational Water Environment. World Health Organization; 2020; WHO/HEP/ECH/WSH/2020.6

[37] Ressom R, Soong FS, Fitzgerald J, Turczynowicz L, El Saadi O, Roder D, et al. Health Effects of Toxic Cyanobacteria (Blue-Green Algae). Australian National Health and Medical Research Council, Looking Glass Press, University of Adelaide; 1994. pp. 1-108. ISBN: 0730822753, 978073 0822752

[38] Hitzfeld BC, Höger SJ, Dietrich DR. Cyanobacterial toxins: Removal during drinking water treatment, and human risk assessment. Environmental Health Perspectives. 2000;**108**:113-122

[39] Fiore M, Cristaldi A, Okatyeva V, Bianco SL, et al. Dietary habits and thyroid cancer risk: A hospital-based case–control study in Sicily (South Italy). Food and Chemical Toxicology. 2020;**146**:111778

[40] Lad A, Breidenbach JD, Su RC, Murray J, Kuang R, et al. As we drink and breathe: Adverse health effects of microcystins and other harmful algal bloom toxins in the liver, gut, lungs and beyond. Life. 2022;**12**(3):418

[41] Weirich CA, Miller TR. Freshwater harmful algal blooms: Toxins and children's health. Current Problems in Pediatric and Adolescent Health Care. 2014;**44**:2-24

[42] Foss AJ, Aubel MT. Using the MMPB technique to confirm microcystin concentrations in water measured by ELISA and HPLC (UV, MS, MS/MS). Toxicon. 2015;**104**:91-101

[43] Chiswell RK, Shaw GR, Eaglesham GK, Smith MJ, Norris RL, Seawright AA, et al. Stability of cylindrospermopsin, the toxin from the

cyanobacterium *Cylindrospermopsis raciborskii*: Effects of pH, temperature and sunlight on decomposition. Environmental Toxicology. 1999;**14**: 155-161

[44] Mokoena MM, Mukhola MS. Current effects of cyanobacteria toxin in water sources and containers in the Hartbeespoort dam area, South Africa. International Journal of Environmental Research and Public Health. 2019;**16**(22): 4468

[45] Spoof L, Błaszczyk A, Meriluoto J, Cegłowska M, Mazur-Marzec H. Structures and activity of new anabaenopeptins produced by Baltic Sea cyanobacteria. Marine Drugs. 2016;**14**:8

[46] Wood SA, Puddick J, Hawes I, Steiner K, Dietrich DR, Hamilton DP. Variability in microcystin quotas during a microcystis bloom in a eutrophic lake. PLoS One. 2021;**16**: e0254967

[47] van Santen JA, Poynton EF, Iskakova D, McMann E, et al. The natural products atlas 2.0: A database of microbially-derived natural products. Nucleic Acids Research. 2022;**50**:D1317-D1323

[48] Codd GA. Cyanobacterial toxins, the perception of water quality, and the prioritisation of eutrophication control. Ecological Engineering. 2000;**16**:51-60

[49] Ibelings BW, Chorus I. Accumulation of cyanobacterial toxins in freshwater "seafood" and its consequences for public health: A review. Environmental Pollutant. 2007; **150**:177-192

[50] Ettoumi A, El Khalloufi F, El Ghazali I, Oudra B, Amrani A, Nasri H, et al. Bioaccumulation of cyanobacterial toxins in aquatic organisms and its consequences for public health. In: Kattel G, editor. Zooplankton and Phyto-Plankton: Types, Characteristics and Ecology. New York: Nova Science Publishers Inc; 2011. pp. 1-34

[51] Hereman TC, do Maria Carmo B-O. Bioaccumulation of microcystins in lettuce. Journal of Phycology. 2012; **48**(6):1535-1537

[52] Anderson DM, Kaoru Y, White AW. Estimated Annual Economic Impacts from Harmful Algal Blooms (HABs) in United States. Woods Hole, MA: Woods Hole Oceanographic Institute Technical Report; 2000

[53] Babica P, Blaha L, Marsalek B. Exploring the natural role of microcystins—A review of effects on photoautotrophic organisms. Journal of Phycology. 2006;**42**(1):9-20

[54] Ku CS, Yang Y, Park Y, Lee J. Health benefits of blue-green algae: Prevention of cardiovascular disease and nonalcoholic fatty liver disease. Journal of Medicinal Food. 2013;**16**(2):103-111. DOI: 10.1089/jmf.2012.2468

[55] Nahin RL, Barnes PM, Stussman BJ, Bloom B. Costs of complementary and alternative medicine (CAM) and frequency of visits to CAM practitioners: United States. National Health Statistics Reports. 2009;**30**:1-14

[56] Roy-Lachapelle A, Solliec M, Bouchard MF, Sauvé S. Detection of cyanotoxins in algae dietary supplements. Toxins (Basel). 2017;**9**(3):76

[57] Smith D. Dietary Supplements Made with Blue-Green Algae Also Contain their Toxins. New York City, US: University of Michigan; Massive Science Inc; 2021. Available from: https://

massivesci.com/articles/cyanobacteria-toxins-blue-green-algae-supplements/

[58] Draisci R, Ferretti E, Palleschi L, Marchiafava C. Identification of anatoxins in blue-green algae food supplements using liquid chromatography-tandem mass spectrometry. Food Additives and Contaminants. 2001;**18**:525-531

[59] Rellán S, Osswald J, Saker M, Gago-Martinez A, Vasconcelos V. First detection of anatoxin-a in human and animal dietary supplements containing cyanobacteria. Food and Chemical Toxicology. 2009;**47**:2189-2195

[60] Dietrich DR, Fischer A, Michel C, Hoeger SJ. Toxin mixture in cyanobacterial blooms—A critical comparison of reality with current procedures employed in human health risk assessment. Advances in Experimental Medicine and Biology. 2008;**619**:885-912

[61] Sivonen K, Niemelä S, Niemi R, Lepistö L, Luoma T, Räsänen L. Toxic cyanobacteria (blue-green algae) in finnish fresh and coastal waters. Hydrobiologia. 1990;**190**:267-275. DOI: 10.1007/BF00008195

[62] Cox PA, Banack SA, Murch SJ, Rasmussen U, Tien G, Bidigare RR, et al. Diverse taxa of cyanobacteria produce β-n-methylamino-l-alanine, a neurotoxic amino acid. Proceedings of the National Academy of Sciences of the United States of America. 2005;**102**:5074-5078

[63] Perumal UE, Sundararaj R. Algae: A potential source to prevent and cure the novel coronavirus – A review. International Journal on Emerging Technologies. 2020;**11**(2):479-483

[64] Ratha SK, Renuka N, Rawat I, Bux F. Prospective options of algae-derived nutraceuticals as supplements to combat COVID-19 and human coronavirus diseases. Nutrition. 2021;**83**:111089. DOI: 10.1016/j.nut.2020.111089

[65] Chia WY, Kok H, Chew KW, Low SS, Show PL. Can algae contribute to the war with Covid-19? Bioengineered. 2021;**12**(1):1226-1237

[66] Facciponte DN, Bough MW, Seidler D, Carroll JL, Ashare A, Andrew AS, et al. Identifying aerosolized cyanobacteria in the human respiratory tract: A proposed mechanism for cyanotoxin-associated diseases. Science of the Total Environment. 2018;**645**:1003-1013

[67] Plaas HE, Paerl HW. Toxic cyanobacteria: A growing threat to water and air quality. Environmental Science & Technology. 2021;**55**(1):44-64

[68] Lim CC, Yoon J, Reynolds K, Gerald LB, Ault AP, Heo S, et al. Harmful algal bloom aerosols and human health. eBioMedicine. 2023;**93**:104604

[69] Reif JS, Stockley N, Harvey K, McFarland M, Gordon SC, Schaefer AM. Symptom frequency and exposure to a cyanobacteria bloom in Florida. Harmful Algae. 2023;**129**:102526

[70] Shi J, Olsonn N, Birbeck J, Pan J, Peraino N, Holen A, et al. Aerosolized cyanobacterial harmful algal bloom toxins: Microcystin congeners quantified in the atmosphere. Environmental Science & Technology. 2023;**57**(51):21801-21814

[71] Schaefer AM, Yrastorza L, Stockley N, Harvey K, Harris N, Grady R, et al. Exposure to microcystin among coastal residents during a cyanobacteria bloom in Florida. Harmful Algae. 2020;**92**:101769

[72] Carmichael WW, Azevedo SM, An JS, Molica RJ, Jochimsen EM, Lau S, et al. Human fatalities from cyanobacteria: Chemical and biological evidence for cyanotoxins. Environmental Health Perspectives. 2001;**109**(7):663-668

[73] Schmidt JR, Wilhelm SW, Boyer GL. The fate of microcystins in the environment and challenges for monitoring. Toxins. 2014;**6**(12): 3354-3387. DOI: 10.3390/toxins6123354

[74] Welker M, Steinberg C. Rates of humic substance photosensitized degradation of microcystin-LR in natural waters. Environmental Science & Technology. 2000;**34**:3415-3419

[75] World Health Organization. Toxic Cyanobacteria in Water: A Guide to their Public Health Consequences, Monitoring and Management. London and New York: Routledge; 1999

[76] Sivonen K. Effects of light, temperature, nitrate, orthophosphate, and bacteria on growth of and hepatotoxin production by *Oscillatoria agardhii* strains. Applied Environmental Microbiology. 1990;**56**:2658-2666

[77] Orr PT, Jones GJ. Relationship between microcystin production and cell division rates in nitrogen-limited *Microcystis aeruginosa* cultures. Limnology and Oceanography. 1998; **43**(7):1604-1614

[78] Rapala J, Robertson A, Negri AP, Berg KA, Tuomi P, Lyra C, et al. First report of saxitoxin in Finnish lakes and possible associated effects on human health. Environmental Toxicology. 2005; **20**(3):331-340

[79] Zurawell RW, Chen H, Burke JM, Prepas EE. Hepatotoxic cyanobacteria: A review of the biological importance of microcystins in freshwater environments. Journal of Toxicology and Environmental Health, Part B. 2005; **8**(1):1-37

[80] Mazur H, Plinski M. Stability of cyanotoxins, microcystin-LR, microcystin-RR and nodularin in seawater and BG-11medium of different salinity. Oceanologia. 2001;**43**:329-339, ISSN:0078-3234

[81] Merel S, Clement M, Thomas O. State of the art on cyanotoxins in water and their behaviour towards chlorine. Toxicon. 2010;**55**:677-691

[82] Carmichael WW. The cyanotoxins. In: Callow JA, editor. Advances in Botanical Research. Vol. 47. London: Academic Press; 1997. pp. 211-255

[83] Duy TN, Lam PKS, Shaw GR, Connell DW. Toxicology and risk assessment of freshwater cyanobacterial (blue-green algal) toxins in water. Reviews of Environmental Contamination and Toxicology. 2000;**163**:113-186

[84] James KJ, Furey A, Sherlock IR, Stack MA, Twohig M, Caudwell FB, et al. Sensitive determination of anatoxin-a, homoanatoxin-a and their degradation products by liquid chromatography with fluorimetric detection. Journal of Chromatography. A. 1998;**798**:147-157

[85] Matsunaga S, Moore RE, Niemczura WP, Carmichael WW. Anatoxin-a(s), a potent anticholinesterase from *Anabaena* flos-aquae. Journal of the American Chemical Society. 1989;**111**:8021-8023

[86] Jones GJ, Negri AP. Persistence and degradation of cyanobacterial paralytic shellfish poisons (PSPs) in freshwaters. Water Research. 1997;**31**: 525-533

[87] World Health Organization. World Health Statistics 2019: Monitoring Health for the SDGs, Sustainable Development Goals. World Health Organization; 2019. p. 120. ISBN: 9789241565707

[88] Höger SJ. Problems during drinking water treatment of cyanobacterial-loaded surface waters: consequences for human health [thesis]. Zur Erlangung des akademischen Grades des Doktors Fakultät für Biologie. Germany: University of Konstanz; 2003

[89] Svirčev V, Krstić S, Miladinov-Mikov M, Baltić V, Vidović M. Freshwater cyanobacterial blooms and primary liver cancer epidemiological studies in Serbia. Journal of Environmental Science and Health. 2009;**C 27**:36-55

[90] Barros MUG, Wilson AE, Leitão JIR, Pereira SP, Buley RP, Fernandez-Figueroa EG, et al. Environmental factors associated with toxic cyanobacterial blooms across 20 drinking water reservoirs in a semi-arid region of Brazil. Harmful Algae. 2019;**86**:128-137

[91] O'Farrell I, Motta C, Forastier M, Polla W, Otaño S, Meichtry N, et al. Ecological meta-analysis of bloom-forming planktonic cyanobacteria in Argentina. Harmful Algae. 2019;**83**:1-13

[92] Rodríguez-Tito JC, Gomez Luna LM, W NN, Alvarez Hubert I. First report on microcystin-LR occurrence in water reservoirs of Eastern Cuba, and environmental trigger factors. Toxins (Basel). 2022;**14**:1-18

[93] Rodas-Pernillo E, Vasquez-Moscoso CA. Evaluación anual del fitoplancton y su respuesta a la calidad de agua en el lago de Amatitlán Guatemala. Ciencia, Tecnología y Salud. 2020;7:54-72

[94] World Health Organization. Cyanobacterial toxins: Microcystin-LR. In: Guidelines for Drinking-Water Quality. Vol. 2. Geneva: World Health Organization; 1998. pp. 95-110

[95] Van Apeldoorn ME, Van Egmond HP, Speijers GJA, Bakker GJI. Toxins of cyanobacteria. Molecular Nutrition & Food Research. 2007;**51**(1):7-60

[96] EDWD. European Drinking Water Directive, 1998/83/EC. Council of the European Union: EDWD; 1998. Available from: http://data.europa.eu/eli/dir/1998/83/oj

[97] Fitzgerald DJ, Cunliffe D, Burch M. Development of health alerts for cyanobacteria and related toxins in drinking water in South Australia. Environmental Toxicology. 1999;**14**:203-209

[98] Azevedo S. New Brazilian regulation for cyanobacteria and cyanotoxins in drinking water. Noosa, Australia: Fifth International Conference on Toxic Cyanobacteria; 2001

[99] Limites de qualite des eaux destinees a la consommation humaine, Decret n° 2001-1220, Annexe I.1. Journal Officiel de la Republique Francaise; LEGIFRANCE; Available from: https://www.legifrance.gouv.fr/eli/decret/2001/12/20/MESX0100156D/jo/texte;2001

[100] Chorus I. Current Approaches to Cyanotoxin Risk Assessment, Risk Management and Regulations in Different Countries. Dessau, Germany: Federal Environmental Agency, (Umweltbundesamt); 2005. p. 122. ISBN 0175-4211

[101] Ministry of Health. Provisional Maximum Acceptable Values for

Cyanotoxins (A3.1.3). New Zealand: Ministry of Health; 2002

[102] NHMRZ/ARMCANZ. Australian Drinking Water Guidelines, Micro-Organism 3: Toxic Algae, Fact Sheets No.17a-17d. Canberra: National Health and Medical Research Council, Agriculture and Resource Management, Australia and New Zealand; 2001

[103] Kouzminov A. New Zealand: Risk assessment, management and regulatory approach for cyanobacteria and cyanotoxins in drinking-water. In: Chorus I, editor. Current Approaches to Cyanotoxin Risk Assessment, Risk Management and Regulations in Different Countries. Berlin: Federal Environmental Agency (Umweltbundesamt); 2005. pp. 93-98

[104] Svrcek C, Smith DW. Cyanobacteria toxins and the current state of knowledge on water treatment options: A review. Journal of Environmental Engineering and Science. 2004;**3**(3):155-185

[105] Fawell JK, James HA. Toxins from Blue-Green Algae: Toxicological Assessment of Anatoxin-a And a Method for its Determination in Reservoir Water. Marlow, UK: FWR Report No. FR0434/DoE 3728, Foundation of Water Research; 1994

[106] Burch M, Humpage A. Australia: Regulation and management of cyanobacteria. In: Chorus I, editor. Current Approaches to Cyanotoxin Risk Assessment, Risk Management and Regulations in Different Countries. Berlin: Federal Environmental Agency; 2005. pp. 9-20

[107] Fawell JK, James CP, James HA. Toxins from Blue-Green Algae: Toxicological Assessment of Microcystin-LR and a Method for its Determination in Water. Medmenham, UK: Water Research Centre; 1994. pp. 1-46

[108] Gilroy DJ, Kauffman KW, Hall RA, Huang X, Chu FS. Assessing potential health risks from microcystin toxins in blue-green algae dietary supplements. Environmental Health Perspectives. 2000;**108**:435-439

[109] World Health Organization. Guidelines for Safe Recreational Water Environments. In: Coastal and Fresh Waters. Volume 1. World Health Organization; 2003. p. 219. ISBN 9241545801

[110] Xie LQ, Xie P, Guo LG, Li L, Miyabara Y, Park HD. Organ distribution and bioaccumulation of microcystins in freshwater fish at different trophic levels from the eutrophic Lake Chaohu, China. Environmental Toxicology. 2005;**20**:293-300

[111] Brasil. Regulation MS N° 2914, "Guidelines for Drinking Water Quality". Official Law Report's; 2011

[112] Bittencourt-Oliveira MC, Piccin-Santos V, et al. Cyanobacteria, microcystins and cylindrospermopsin in public drinking supply reservoirs of Brazil. Anais da Academia Brasileira de Ciências. 2013;**86**(1):297-310

[113] Brasil. PORTARIA GM/MS No 888, de 4 de maio de 2021. Brasília, DF: Ministry of Health; 2021

[114] Svirčev Z, Drobac D, Tokodi N, Đenić D, Simeunović J, Hiskia A, et al. Lessons from the Užice case: How to complement analytical data; chapter 31. In: Meriluoto J, Spoof L, Codd GA, editors. Handbook of Cyanobacterial Monitoring and Cyanotoxin Analysis. Wiley publisher; 2016. Print ISBN:

9781119068686 |Online ISBN: 9781119068761

[115] Tanber G. Toxin Leaves 500,000 in Northwest Ohio without Drinking Water. London: Reuters; 2014

[116] Hernandez BY, Zhu X, Nagata M, Loo L, Chan O, Wong LL. Cyanotoxin exposure and hepatocellular carcinoma. Toxicology. 2023;**487**:153470

[117] Ritchie H, Spooner F, Roser M. Sanitation. Our World in Data; 2019. Available from: https://ourworldindata.org/sanitation

[118] Stanaway JD, Afshin A, Gakidou E, et al. Global, regional, and national comparative risk assessment of 84 behavioural, environmental and occupational, and metabolic risks or clusters of risks for 195 countries and territories, 1990–2017: A systematic analysis for the global burden of disease study 2017. The Lancet. 2018; **392**(10159):1923-1994

[119] Simeunović J, Svirčev Z, Krstić S, Lazić L. Occurrence of cyanobacterial blooms in Vojvodina water ecosystems. Geographica Pannonica. 2005;**9**:13-19

[120] Teixera M, Costa M, Carvalho V, Pereira M, Hage E. Gastroenteritis epidemic in the area of the Itaparica dam, Bahia, Brazil. Bulletin of the Pan American Health Organiyation. 1993;**27**: 244-253

[121] Westrick JA. Everything a manager should know about algal toxins but was afraid to ask. Journal of American Water Works Association. 2003;**95**:26-34

[122] Höger SJ, Shaw G, Hitzfeld BC, Dietrich DR. Occurrence and elimination of cyanobacterial toxins in two Australian drinking water treatment plants. Toxicon. 2004;**43**:639-649

[123] Tisdale ES. Combating tastes in West Virginia water supplies in 1930. Journal AWWA. 1931;**23**(9):1357-1365

[124] Bourke ATC, Hawes RB, Neilson A, Stallman ND. An outbreak of hepato-enteritis (the Palm Island mystery disease) possibly caused by algal intoxication. Toxicon. 1983;**3**:45-48

[125] Miller AP, Tisdale ES. Epidemic of intestinal disorders in Charleston, West Virginia, occurring simultaneously with unprecedented water supply conditions. American Journal of Public Health. 1931; **21**:198-200

[126] Zilberg B. Gastroenteritis in Salisbury European children—A five-year study. Central African Journal of Medicine. 1966;**12**(9):164-168

[127] Humpage AR, Rositano J, Breitag AH, Brown R, Baler PD, Nicholson WC, et al. Paralytic shellfish poisons from Australian cyanobacterial blooms. Australian Journal of Marine & Freshwater Research. 1994;**45**:761-777

[128] Francis G. Poisonous Australian lake. Nature. 1878;**18**:11-12

[129] Steyn DG. Poisoning of animals by algae on dams and pans. Farming in South Africa. 1943;**18**:489-492

[130] Mez K, Hanselmann K, Naegeli H, Preisig HR. Protein phosphatase-inhibiting activity in cyanobacteria from alpine lakes in Switzerland. Phycologia. 1996;**35**:133-139

[131] Cronberg G, Gieske A, Martins E, Nengu PJ, Stenstrom I-M. Hydrobiological studies of the Okavango Delta and Kwando/Linyanti/Chobe river, Botswana. In: Surface Water Quality Analysis. Vol. 27. Botswana Notes and Records; 1995;**27**:151-226

[132] Mahmood NA, Carmichael WW, Pfahler D. Anticholinesterase poisonings in dogs from a cyanobacterial (blue-green algae) bloom dominated by *Anabaena flosaquae*. American Journal of Veterinary Research. 1988;**49**(4): 500-503

[133] Kann J, Falter CM. Development of toxic blue-green algal blooms in black lake, Kootenai County, Idaho. Lake and Reservoir Management. 2009;**3**(1): 99-108. DOI: 10.1080/0743814870 9354765

[134] Van der Merwe D, Sebbag L, Nietfeld JC, Aubel MT, Foss A, Carney E. Investigation of a *Microcystis aeruginosa* cyanobacterial freshwater harmful algal bloom associated with acute microcystin toxicosis in a dog. Journal of Veterinary Diagnostic Investigation. 2012;**24**: 679-687

[135] Backer LC, Landsberg JH, Miller M, Keel K, Taylor TK. Canine cyanotoxin poisonings in the United States (1920s-2012): Review of suspected and confirmed cases from three data sources. Toxins (Basel). 2013;**5**:1597-1628. DOI: 10.3390/toxins5091597

[136] Botes DP, Wessels PL, Kruger H, Runnegar MTC, Santikarn S, Smith RJ, et al. Structural studies on cyanoginosins-LR, YR, YA, and YM, peptide toxins from *Microcystis aeruginosa*. Journal of The Chemical Society-perkin Transactions. 1985;**1**: 2747-2748

[137] Falconer IR, Beresford AM, Runnegar MTC. Evidence of liver damage by toxin from a bloom of the blue-green alga, *Microcystis aeruginosa*. The Medical Journal of Australia. 1983;**1**: 511-514

[138] Yu S-Z. Drinking water and primary liver cancer. In: Tang ZY, Wu MC, Xia SS, editors. Primary Liver Cancer. New York: China Academic Publishers; 1989. pp. 30-37

[139] Yu S-Z. Primary prevention of hepatocellular carcinoma. Journal of Gastroenterology and Hepatology. 1995; **10**:674-682

[140] Sivonen K, Jones G. Cyanobacterial toxins. In: ChorusI BJ, editor. Toxic Cyanobacteria in Water: A Guide to Public Health Significance, Monitoring and Management. London: E&FN Spon; 1999. pp. 41-111

[141] de la Cruz AA, Antoniou MG, Hiskia A, Pelaez M, Song W, O'Shea KE, et al. Can we effectively degrade microcystins? Implications on human health. Anti-Cancer Agents in Medical Chemistry. 2011;**11**:19-37

[142] Svirčev Z, Drobac D, Tokodi N, Lužanin Z, Munjas AM, Nikolin B, et al. Epidemiology of cancers in Serbia and possible connection with cyanobacterial blooms. Journal of Environmental Science and Health Part C Environmental Carcinogenesis & Ecotoxicology Reviews. 2014;**32**(4): 319-337

[143] Wert EC, Rosario-Ortiz FL. Intracellular organic matter from cyanobacteria as a precursor for carbonaceous and nitrogenous disinfection byproducts. Environmental Science & Technology. 2013;**47**: 6332-6340

[144] Mohamed ZA, Deyab MA, Abou-Dobara MI, El-Sayed AK, El-Raghi WM. Occurrence of cyanobacteria and microcystin toxins in raw and treated waters of the Nile river, Egypt: Implication for water treatment and human health. Environmental Science and Pollution Research. 2015;**22**: 11716-11727

[145] Carmichael WW. Assessment of Blue-Green Algal Toxins in Raw and Finished Drinking Water. Denver, Colorado: AWWA Research Foundation; 2001. pp. 1-179

[146] Zamyadi A, MacLeod S, Fan Y, McQuaid N, Dorner S, Sauvé S, et al. Toxic cyanobacterial breakthrough and accumulation in a drinking water plant: A monitoring and treatment challenge. Water Research. 2012;**46**(5): 1511-1523

[147] Pietsch J, Bornmann K, Schmidt W. Relevance of intra- and extracellular cyanotoxins for drinking water treatment. Acta Hydrochimica et Hydrobiologica. 2002;**30**(1):7-15

[148] Wang H, Ho L, Lewis DM, Brookes JD, Newcombe G. Discriminating and assessing adsorption and biodegradation removal mechanisms during granular activated carbon filtration of microcystin toxins. Water Research. 2007;**41**(18):4262-4270

[149] Peng Y, Yang X, Ren B, Zhang Z, Deng X, Yin W, et al. Algae removal characteristics of the ultrasonic radiation enhanced drinking water treatment process. Journal of Water Process Engineering. 2023;**55**:104154

[150] Bourne DG, Blakeley RL, Riddles P, Jones GJ. Biodegradation of the cyanobacterial toxin microcystin-LR in natural water and biologically active slow sand filters. Water Research. 2006; **40**(6):1294-1302

[151] Saito T, Okano K, Park HD, Itayama T, Inamori Y, Neilan BA, et al. Detection and sequencing of the microcystin LR-degrading gene, mlrA, from new bacteria isolated from Japanese lakes. FEMS Microbiology Letters. 2003;**229**:271-276

[152] Manage PM, Edwards C, Singh BK, Lawton LA. Isolation and identification of novel microcystin degrading bacteria. Applied Environmental Microbiology. 2009;**75**:6924-6928

[153] Welgama A. Novel Bacterial Strains Clear Algal Toxins from Drinking Water. Society for General Microbiology. Rockville, Maryland: Science Daily; 2009

[154] Stumpf RP, Davis TW, Wynne TT, Graham JL, Loftin KA, Johengen TH, et al. Challenges for mapping cyanotoxin patterns from remote sensing of cyanobacteria. Harmful Algae. 2016;**54**: 160-173. DOI: 10.1016/j.hal.2016.01.005

[155] Kutser T. Passive optical remote sensing of cyanobacteria and other intense phytoplankton blooms in coastal and inland waters. International Journal of Remote Sensing. 2009;**30**(17): 4401-4425

[156] Tilzer MM. Light-dependence of photosynthesis and growth in cyanobacteria: Implications for their dominance in eutrophic lakes. New Zealand Journal of Marine and Freshwater Research. 1987;**21**(3): 401-412

[157] Paerl HW, Fulton RS, Moisander PH, Dyble J. Harmful freshwater algal blooms, with an emphasis on cyanobacteria. Scientific World Journal. 2001;**1**:76-113

[158] Huisman J, Sharples J, Stroom JM, Visser PM, Kardinaal WEA, Verspagen JMH, et al. Changes in turbulent mixing shift competition for light between phytoplankton species. Ecology. 2004;**85**:2960-2970

[159] Kohoutek J, Babica P, Bláha L, et al. A novel approach for monitoring of cyanobacterial toxins: Development and

evaluation of the passive sampler for microcystins. Analytical and Bioanalytical Chemistry. 2008;**390**: 1167-1172

[160] Kohoutek J, Maršálek B, Bláha L. Evaluation of the novel passive sampler for cyanobacterial toxins microcystins under various conditions including field sampling. Analytical and Bioanalytical Chemistry. 2010;**397**:823-828

[161] Jaša L, Sadílek J, Kohoutek J, Straková L, Maršálek B, Babica P. Application of passive sampling for sensitive time-integrative monitoring of cyanobacterial toxins microcystins in drinking water treatment plants. Water Research. 2019;**153**:108-120

[162] Loaiza-González JM, Rubio-Clemente A, Peñuela GA. Cyanotoxin monitoring and detection using passive sampling application. Water, Air, and Soil Pollution. 2024;**235**:423

[163] Cunningham BR, Wharton RE, Lee C, Mojica MA, Krajewski LC, et al. Measurement of microcystin activity in human plasma using immunocapture and protein phosphatase inhibition assay. Toxins. 2022;**14**:813

[164] Yuan M, Carmichael WW, Hilborn ED. Microcystin analysis in human sera and liver from human fatalities in Caruaru, Brazil 1996. Toxicon. 2006;**48**:627-640

[165] Wharton RE, Ojeda-Torres G, Cunningham B, Feyereisen MC, Hill KL, et al. Quantification of microcystin-LR in human urine by immunocapture liquid chromatography tandem mass spectrometry. Chemical Research in Toxicology. 2018;**31**:898-903

[166] Palagama DSW, Baliu-Rodriguez D, Lad A, Levison BS, Kennedy DJ, Haller ST, et al. Development and applications of solid-phase extraction and liquid chromatography-mass spectrometry methods for quantification of microcystins in urine, plasma, and serum. Journal of Chromatography. A. 2018;**1573**:66-77

[167] Hilborn ED, Carmichael WW, Yuan M, Azevedo SMFO. A simple colorimetric method to detect biological evidence of human exposure to microcystins. Toxicon. 2005;**46**:218-221

[168] Carmichael WW, Boyer GL. Health impacts from cyanobacteria harmful algae blooms: Implications for the north American Great Lakes. Harmful Algae. 2016;**54**:194-212

[169] Rankin KA, Alroy KA, Kudela RM, Oates SC, Murray MJ, Miller MA. Treatment of cyanobacterial (microcystin) toxicosis using oral cholestyramine: Case report of a dog from Montana. Toxins (Basel). 2013; **5**(6):1051-1063

[170] IANAS. Water Quality in the Americas. Risks and Opportunities. 1st ed. Mexico: IANAS & UNESCO; 2019. p. 626

[171] Rashidi H, Baulch H, Gill A, Bharadwaj L, Bradford L. Monitoring, managing, and communicating risk of harmful algal blooms (HABs) in recreational resources across Canada. Environmental Health Insights. 2021;**15**: 11786302211014401